Read This
Before Medical School

How to Study Smarter and Live Better While Excelling in Class and on Your USMLE or COMLEX Board Exams

Indies United Publishing House, LLC

INDIES UNITED PUBLISHING HOUSE, LLC
P.O. BOX 3071
QUINCY, IL 62305-3071
www.indiesunited.net

About the Authors

Chase DiMarco: Chase is an MS, MBA-HA and MD/Ph.D-candidate. He is the Founder and educator at FreeMedEd, which he began in 2014 to consolidate free educational resources for his classmates. He also hosts the Medical Mnemonist Podcast, is Chief Development Officer at InsideTheBoards, and CEO of MedMatch Externships clinical rotations service. He has explored many facets of medical education, the psychology of learning, and accelerated learning techniques. As an average student, it wasn't until after he had attained graduate education that he learned to implement accelerated learning and educational efficiency. Now, with a passion to make studying easier for all students and bring great educational resources to the masses, he has worked to compile some of the top literature out there on Educational Psychology, Academic Medicine, and Memory.

Greg Rodden: Greg is a pediatrics resident in Austin, TX, and founder/host of the Med School Phys podcast. When he's not being a doctor for kids, he tries to stay happy and healthy by listening to podcasts & audiobooks on long walks, doting on his dog, and leisurely dining with his wife. Greg is dedicated to providing high-quality medical education to anyone who is willing to learn.

Theodore X. O'Connell: Ted is a family physician, educator, and author of many popular books, including the Crush Step series and the USMLE Step Secrets series. He is the founding director of the Family Medicine residency training program at Kaiser Permanente Napa-Solano and is an Associate Clinical Professor in the Department of Family and Community Medicine at the UC San Francisco School of Medicine. Dr. O'Connell is passionate about helping the next generation of physicians become successful, both as clinicians and as future professionals who can confidently navigate medical culture. He hopes his collective works will help cultivate outstanding physicians.

Table of Contents

PREFACE

How to Use this Book

First off, thank you for choosing to read this book. You will not regret it. We will provide you with a vast array of suggestions for studying, tools we personally used to excel in medical school, tips for self-improvement, and guidance to keep you on the path to success. This is not simply a "medical study resource," but rather it is a guidebook filled with wisdom and pearls about everything related to your future career in medicine.

Some books will teach you how to make flashcards, some have tips for test-day, while others focus on efficiency and scheduling. This book incorporates all of those topics, and more! To scratch the surface, we will give you a tried and true approach to tackle board exam-style questions, tips to accelerate your learning speed, and advice on how to use flashcards, while also covering topics like burnout prevention during this challenging time in your life. There is currently NO OTHER resource that offers this much information, assembled together in one place, and without the fluff.

If you are already aware of some of the concepts discussed throughout, you've got a big headstart and we will help you to optimize your existing strategies. If it all seems new, don't worry. We'll explain everything in detail and provide concrete examples to help you get started. Discovering these kinds of learning techniques and strategies is probably best before you start medical school, but even if you've already begun classes, don't be discouraged. There's no time like the present!

We aim to provide you with a no-nonsense guide to success in medical school and beyond. As such, we have researched, analyzed, and synthesized dozens of top-rated books, hundreds of research papers, and years of experience in medicine and education to create an excellent product. It would be impossible for us to perform a systematic review of every subject we cover, but we gave it our best shot.

Regardless, it's healthy to question everything you see, hear, and read these days (without being a contrarian). Remain reasonable and open-minded if you encounter something new here. We urge you to experiment, record the results, reassess, rinse and repeat. When you've found something that works, we urge you to engage in Deliberate Practice to maximize your results. But let's not get ahead of ourselves; this is just the introduction.

If you have already skimmed through the Table of Contents, you may have noticed the overarching structure of this book, which is broken up into four main parts:

Part 1: Overview of Study Skills & Work-Life Balance
Part 2: Test Preparation and Exam Day
Part 3: Accelerated Learning and Mnemonics
Part 4: Self-Assessment

Considering how much content we cover, you should not feel obligated to follow along section-by-section. Some areas may be of greater relevance to you right now, while others can take a back seat. **Jump from section to section as needed**. We thank you for your support and hope you enjoy the book.

Occam's Razor vs. Hickam's Dictum

Advising learners on something as complicated as medical education is tricky. No two students are the same, so we need to be flexible when providing advice about the approach to learning, the best resources, and the study habits to reinforce. Ultimately, you have to find what works for you. One topic might be learned best by a familiar or obvious method, while another lesson may require uncomfortable or outside-the-box thinking. This is a sort of *Occam's Razor vs. Hickam's Dictum* situation for your medical education where the simplest solution is the best... until it isn't.

Herein, we attempt to provide a wealth of different recommendations and educational strategies that you can explore. It will require you to spend a little more time upfront to determine what works best for you. A word of caution: you will be tempted to first choose the method that you LIKE best, but keep in mind that it may not be the method that WORKS best for you. This is where an open mind and honest self-assessment will really show their value. Throughout the text, we encourage regular self-assessment and we provide plenty of concrete examples to see how you can gauge your performance.

A Doctor's Timeline

Before diving into how to thrive in medical school, we should probably lay out the timeline for you. What will your life look like when going through your medical training? Obviously, there will be variations on this theme, but here's the basic timeline for someone who goes straight from undergrad to attending physician:

Year 1	Spring	Finish Undergrad
	Fall	Start MS1 - Preclinical studies (basic sciences)
Year 2	Fall	Start MS2 - Preclinical studies (basic sciences)
	Spring	USMLE Step 1 or COMLEX Level 1 - Multiple choice exam
Year 3	Fall	Start MS3 - Clinical rotations
	Spring	USMLE CS or COMLEX PE - Standardized patient encounters
		USMLE Step 2 or COMLEX Level 2 - Multiple choice exam
Year 4	Fall	Start MS4 - Clinical rotations
		ERAS - Submit applications to residency programs
	Spring	Residency Match Day
		Finish Medical School
Year 5	PGY1	Intern year
		USMLE Step 3 or COMLEX Level 3 - Multiple choice exam
Year 6	PGY2	
Year 7+	PGY3+	Residency length depends on the program
...		
Optional	Fellowship	Typically 1-3 years of subspecialty training
...		
Goal	Attending Physician	

Don't freak out after seeing this! Yes, you've got a long way to go, but if you're passionate about patient care and medical science, you belong on this path.

Other Career Options

Most doctors begin their journey of medical education in the same way. We worked hard during college and stressed out about getting into medical school. Then, we worked hard and stressed out about passing boards and getting a good residency. Some repeat the cycle for fellowship. And then we stress out about our patients, our business, and our administrative duties. While life in medicine is rewarding, it can also be very stressful!

Most doctors do not seriously consider anything other than the default pathway into clinical practice. If this is your goal, great. If you are unsure, also great. Why? Because there is a significant need for highly skilled and educated professionals both in clinical practice and outside of the hospital. If you have never been educated on the other options, or you were never taught the skills related to success in fields outside of medicine, you may feel like you have no other choice. That couldn't be further from the truth.

Within the confines of this book, we cannot comprehensively teach about all of the important skills for leadership, business, and education related to medicine (and other professions), but we will offer solid advice from trusted resources for your own exploration. If you're unsure about where you want to take your MD or DO degree, just take a moment to peek outside of the bubble. You can start with a website like Docjobs.com. Just becoming aware of the other options available to you can significantly alleviate the stress you may be feeling.

PART 1: OVERVIEW OF STUDY SKILLS & WORK-LIFE BALANCE

Time in the Classroom

"Education is what survives when what has
been learned has been forgotten."
B.F. Skinner

Pre-Test: On a scale of 1-7 (1 = never and 7 = always) rate these questions.

#	Question/Statement	SCORE
1	I come to class prepared each day.	/7
2	I participate in class frequently and effectively.	/7
3	I communicate questions clearly to the instructor and to my classmates.	/7
4	I listen actively, try to formulate questions to topics being discussed, and reflect on these ideas.	/7
5	I know how to communicate with my instructor out of class and the best time to do so.	/7
6	I know the resources my school has available, and how to access them.	/7
	TOTAL	/42

This section was particularly difficult to write for a general audience, as the structure of classes varies greatly across educational institutions. Some students are adamant about attending every lecture, extracurricular activity, and guest speaker available to them. Others prefer to focus on self-study while attending as few classes as possible.

Generally, lecturers will speak at around 100 words per minute, often less. As you will see in the Accelerated Learning section, that is unbearably slow for some students. Though there are pros and cons to attending vs. not, both approaches can be successful. The utility of attending live lectures is determined by a host of factors, but the one you have control over is your personal preference (and hopefully your school doesn't have an attendance policy).

Your time is valuable. Period. If you don't get much out of class, do your own thing and don't feel obligated to listen when you're there. If you derive greater benefit from class study than personal study, find ways to get the most out of class. This includes regular/active participation, asking well-constructed and properly-timed questions, having a detailed knowledge of your academic schedule, and knowing about the particular resources provided by your school.

> *Note from Greg: During the first year of medical school, I tried my best to pay attention in class, but I slowly learned that I could not maximize my time there. Eventually, I found it best to tune into one or two lectures per day and then plug in headphones to study on my own for the remaining lectures.*

Class Participation

Do you arrive to class prepared, or do you just *wing it*? Do you download, print, and pre-read the syllabus and all other course content before the first day of class? Or do you wait for the instructor to point out what they think is important? There are many ways to be prepared for class, whether it be your first day or your last semester. Though Wifi and digital resources make it increasingly easy to have the proper materials with you at all times, mental preparation can be a little more ambiguous.

Many Americans actually *fear of public speaking* more than death [1], and class participation can feel very similar. We may think, "What if they think I'm stupid for asking that question?" The best response is, "So what?" In all likelihood, your classmates won't spend their day judging your every move; they have their own issues to deal with. But if this is a real concern for you, the Anxiety and Depression Association of America has some tips [2]:

1) Focus on the contribution to your audience, not yourself.
2) Focus on calming and reassuring images instead of dreading what may go wrong.
3) Point out and eliminate negative thoughts.
4) Use calming practices such as deep breathing, yoga, and meditation.
5) Prepare ahead of time and practice.
6) Connect with your audience.
7) Confident posture! External confidence can help your internal confidence.
8) Give up perfection. Accept mistakes and learn from them.

Equating a phobia of public speaking to asking a quick question in class may seem a little extreme, but it can produce significant anxiety in the moment. Try using the recommendations above if you're struggling. Learning to be relaxed and prepared can help prevent the fidgeting, sweating, stammering, and shaking presentation that everyone fears. Believe us, we've been there.

One other factor that will help the nervous public speaker is to prepare your question or comment properly. Blurting out every thought or question that pops into your head doesn't make you an active participant, it makes you an *ask-hole*. On the other hand, you may have a very valuable question that could benefit the whole class. How do you decide?

If you prepared for the class ahead of time, you might have a helpful question that is not covered by the lecture materials. Even a cursory glance at the material may save you from posing an obvious question/comment that is answered by the next slide. Your next step, if applicable, could be a quick internet search while the lecture continues on. This can answer most questions without disrupting the class. In medical school, the more important questions for you and your classmates will usually revolve around concepts.

Some subjects, like physiology or pharmacology, require a lot of background conceptual knowledge. So, the questions posed in these areas are not always easily answered by a quick internet search. If you are prepared for class and still are not sure what is going on, it may be a good time to raise those four fingers and a thumb. Chances are if you prepared and still don't get it, then there are plenty of other people who are lost. This would be a shortcoming on the part of the presenter, not the student.

If the answer provided by the instructor is not sufficient, try to rephrase your question in a very direct and specific manner. Be clear. Be tactful. Be respectful both to the lecturer and other students. Give examples, if possible, because it is very hard for most instructors to answer an overgeneralized or vague question in the moment. When in-class questions are used properly, you can be sure your classmates will appreciate the effort.

Sometimes you cannot ask a question in the moment, so you will have to look it up at home, send an email, or ask at the next class. **Don't accept not knowing.** Many topics in medicine will build upon themselves [3], so you should do your very best to quench your thirst for knowledge.

Now that we have a guide to self-confidence, and knowing how to ask proper questions, what is the best way to proactively set up your environment in class for successful learning? First, you don't need to sit in the front row to make the best of your situation, but the back of the room is not a great choice for those who want to participate. Sit close enough that you can clearly hear the lecturer and see any of the visuals used for instruction. This also helps your questions to be easily heard. If your class has windows, you may want to account for the time of day and the effect of glare on screens. Also, it's not a bad idea to have a buffer seat between you and your friends, if at all possible, just to avoid distractions. Last, if you plan to do your own thing during class, consider sitting in the back so your computer screen doesn't distract the people who sit behind you.

Effective Use of Your Professor's Time

Every educator is different. Some teachers are very clear about office hours, their expectations, if they allow extra credit or not, etc. **Respect their time and their system**. Just like you, your instructors are busy people. They have family obligations, research projects, and clinical duties to worry about. Feel free to jump ahead to the Emotional Intelligence section later in Part 1 if you need a better understanding of what *a mile in their shoes* feels like.

Once you understand your instructor's schedule and willingness to assist outside of class, set up a meeting with them. Bring a clear list of questions if that will help. At the very least, setting up an appointment to clarify confusing material before an exam - or going over questions after the exam - is a great way to benefit from their expertise.

> ***Email Template:*** *"Dr./Professor _____, I seem to be having trouble with (subject, concept, process). I think at this point I may need more direct guidance here. May I schedule an appointment to discuss this with you? Perhaps if I show you (what I'm doing, how I'm thinking), you might be able to help me understand the topic better? I believe that (time A, B, or C) could work for both of us. Which would you prefer?"*

The email template above is short, direct, and polite. When you communicate this clearly and deliberately, the instructor will have a better idea of how to prepare for the meeting and where they may need to tweak their existing materials. If the one-on-one meeting doesn't help, ask them for another resource (or even an old exam). Most instructors are happy to provide assistance to motivated and courteous students, so don't worry about being a burden to them.

Side note: if an instructor is generous enough to agree to a meeting or mentoring session with you, you would be unwise to arrive late to (or miss) the appointment. This is valuable time and should be treated as such. Some instructors might opt to arrange group sessions if the topic is commonly misunderstood, but this will vary based on the school, topic, and instructor.

Using School Resources

If you come from a small school with few resources, much of this section may not apply. Or there may be abundant resources at your disposal. Either way, **use what you're given!**

The Academic Affairs Office, Student Organizations, Learning Centers, and a host of other resources are at your fingertips. You are paying for these services through your tuition anyway; why let them go to waste? Research databases, online textbooks, and question banks are offered nearly universally, even at smaller schools. Explore what's available to you and experiment to see what works.

One obvious resource is the school library. A library isn't just a place to check out books and quietly study. Most librarians have a gold mine of information that they are eager to share. Beyond finding (e)books, journal articles, pages on the school website, audiobooks, and videos, school librarians can also help you to access resources your school doesn't directly offer.

School counselors are also an underused resource at most campuses. You may have different types of counselors for different needs, but most often you can seek help with occupational guidance, managing life stressors, and emotional support. With burnout percentages running as high as 50% in some studies [4], these staff members should probably be seeing every student.

The negative stigma of seeking social or emotional support is very strong in males and type A personalities (which is common among medical students). But the climate in medicine is changing [5]. There is no reason to fear using these services. We will also cover ways to manage and prevent burnout in several upcoming sections.

Though all U.S. schools offer disability services, many students don't think to use them. That makes sense at first glance... until you realize that somewhere between 5% and 20% of students are reported to have some sort of learning disability [6,7]. Many will go into higher education without ever knowing it.

The stigma of being labeled with a "learning disability" can also be difficult to overcome. We are not taught much about these disorders as a part of the standard medical curriculum. If you are having difficulty with your coursework or suspect that something might be *off*, explore the issue and make use of your available resources. Unfortunately, many students wait until they have repeated issues on exams to seek help.

Studies Outside of the Classroom

Pre-Test: On a scale of 1-7 (1 = never and 7 = always) rate these questions.

#	Question/Statement	SCORE
1	I have designed and created an area designated for efficient studying.	/7
2	I have the tools and materials needed to optimize my study sessions.	/7
3	I reviewed all the material I studied yesterday in under 1 hour (from initial review) and will review it again today.	/7
4	I have a prioritized to-do list of all activities I must complete (daily, weekly, etc.).	/7
5	I am aware of methods and procedures to monitor my study sessions for efficiency and also to locate weaknesses.	/7
6	I write down words and topics I am unfamiliar with to review later.	/7
	TOTAL	/42

The home (or outside the classroom environment) is where medical students spend the majority of their study time. Even for those who attend every class, guest lecture, and extracurricular, the majority of your deep learning will happen on your own time.

Most of us know that it's tough to absorb classroom instruction in real-time. Most medical schools still provide instruction in the old school way: hours of lectures and hundreds of PowerPoint slides a day. It's no wonder that students - even those seeking professional degrees - will socialize, check social media, watch cat videos, or even sleep in the classroom... guilty. Don't be that person.

Modern students tend to prefer shorter-class lengths that are spread out, as opposed to all at once [8]. Some studies show a decrease in on-task behavior as lectures drone on [9], while others show a "waxing and waning" of attention spans [10]. Even college students' attention span is said to decrease after just 10-15 minutes of a lecture, though this assertion is opposed in more recent research [10].

Medical education has lagged behind most other industries by remaining teacher-centered instead of student-centered. This leads to extra strain on the student, more work for the instructor, and likely contributes to burnout, anxiety, and depression [11,12].

Some schools have modernized in recent years, adding Problem-based learning (PBL) and pre-recorded lectures to their curriculum. These options reduce the time-wasting redundancies of lecturers preparing and presenting the same material time and time again. Accelerated video playback speeds help to limit the monotony of long speeches and boring presentation slides. And using screen capture software allows for an easier creation of study notes and flashcards. All of these features allow for increased student autonomy.

Regardless of whether your medical curriculum is up-to-date or old school, you will find yourself spending huge chunks of each day studying alone or in a group. To make the best use of this time, we will provide some often-overlooked adjustments to your study environment that will help you to work more efficiently.

As a quick caveat, our Accelerated Learning section will have study hacks from former medical students who only studied a few hours a week while traveling around the world, memory techniques from mnemonists who have won memory championships, and efficient study habits from accelerated learning instructors who have successfully taught these skills to thousands of learners.

Creating the Ultimate Study Environment

Ergonomic Design

When creating your study area, the first thing likely on your mind is what hardware to consider. The most obvious items would be your desk, chair, and computer or other electronic devices. However, there are many other little additions that can decrease clutter, reduce mental strain, and challenge you in positive ways. For the big three, the most common issues concerning these items are cost, size, and features. But many of us are more swayed by the features we *want* rather than focusing on the features we actually *need*.

Ergonomics may be a term considered synonymous with comfort, but it is much more than that. Many products use the term without putting any consideration into what it really means. Ergonomics is "the science of designing the job to fit the worker, rather than physically forcing the worker's body to fit the job" [13]. The CDC recognizes that many musculoskeletal injuries – and their negative effects on the economy – could be prevented by ergonomic designs [14].

So, ergonomic design is an important consideration for any job, including the job of a student. It aims to create tools that help to prevent musculoskeletal issues that are typically caused by repetitive tasks. The U.S. Navy even released a document recommending a list of adjustment features required for ergonomic chairs [15]. Though most commercial office chairs now fit the requirements, this doesn't mean that every chair will fit *you*. We are all built differently, so a bit of trial and error may be required.

Desk adjustability features are similarly important. Adjustable and standing desks are all the rage, and many hospitals have adopted the use of adjustable tabletop desks, as well as the computer on wheels (COW). Standing desks are said to have many potential health benefits (although this is still unproven [16]), while not necessarily being detrimental to employee task-management [17]. In fact, Dr. Michael Greger of NutritionFacts.org and author of *How Not to Die*

17

(to be discussed in the nutrition section) holds all of his meetings while on a treadmill desk.

If money is a concern (as it often is for medical students) there are plenty of DIY options to achieve similar results. Even a simple project with PVC pipes, a cardboard box, and some duct tape will get the job done. If your creativity is failing at the moment, pulling up a DIY video could offer some insight.

Though sitting vs. standing may be up for debate, there is little argument that having the option to go from sitting to standing, or vice versa, is not a bad thing. When it comes to your posture, having options and adjusting position as needed can reduce the strain on the large joints vulnerable to aches and pains.

Also, on the subject of body posture and extended times at a desk, make sure to relax your eyes and stretch your muscles from time to time. The American Optometric Association recommends using the 20-20-20 Rule to prevent eye strain: take a 20-second break every 20 minutes to look at something else 20 feet away [18]. To help prevent muscle strain you can search "computer stretches" or "desk stretches" as well.

Accessories

Now that you are in a comfortable position, let's talk about study accessories. When considering desk accessories, **minimalism is key**. You don't need *more* accessories, you just need the ones that serve important functions for your workflow.

This is a good time to mention that, as a medical student, a resident, and a full-fledged attending, you will be moving your stuff frequently. Weigh the pros and cons of each item. Do you really want to take it with you when you move? Or can you purchase a new one at your next location? Anyone who has moved multiple times will endorse this kind of thinking.

A combination office-organizer and adjustable monitor stand is a great multi-purpose tool. You can purchase low-profile desk caddies that stick to your external monitor. There are many new and improved designs, so doing a quick online search for "desk caddy," "office organizer," or "DIY office" may save you some time (compared to shopping in brick & mortar stores).

Another helpful tool is a whiteboard to organize your thoughts and do-to lists. Some of these may later be transferred to a to-do app, but there's nothing like being able to see everything on your plate at one time. If you're feeling creative, you can even DIY a whiteboard using markable glass or hardboard panels.

Last, let's bring our attention to noise pollution. There has been a lot of research in the past few years regarding noise pollution in cities, including its effects on alertness, mental health, and other health concerns. There are even studies that show noise pollution can even produce enough stress to raise your blood pressure, which is a known risk factor for cardiovascular events [19].

From a macroscopic view, the biggest thing you can do to avoid noise pollution is to choose a quiet neighborhood. This peace of mind may be worth the extra rent. Asking a local friend, family member, or real-estate agent could help you narrow your search for the ideal living space. Many of us are not squared away financially in medical school, so you may not be able to find a quiet place that's in your budget.

But even if you're not in the best macro-environment, you should still be able to optimize your study micro-environment. Let's consider options that will help to limit the effects of noise pollution on your studies. First and foremost: headgear. People rave about noise-canceling headsets that cost several hundred dollars, debate the use of in-ear vs. over-ear options, and cherry-pick anecdotes that confirm their previously held beliefs. At the end of the day, it's about personal preference.

A simple pair of gun store earmuffs can be highly effective. If they can block out gunshots at the shooting range, they can do a pretty good job of blocking out your neighbor's barking dogs. We've found that this simple, cheap option can work better than the expensive noise-canceling headphones. Even a pair of foam ear-plugs can work. If you have issues with cerumen impaction or ear infections, this may not be the best idea.

Although noise pollution is something we, as students, generally try to avoid, there is an argument against doing so at times. If you fixate on getting your environment absolutely silent, you will just be wasting valuable time [20]. Whether we like it or not, noise is everywhere, and the last thing we need is to develop anxiety about finding the best and quietest spot to study. Good thing we can carry around our noise-reducing headgear wherever we go, right?

An interesting approach that was discussed in the book *Medical School 2.0* is to PURPOSELY study in a noisy environment. This may not work for all students or situations. However, Dr. Larson claims that studying in noisy coffee shops helped him to develop greater focus while studying and taking exams. If you study like a Zen master in a busy coffee shop, you may not be too disturbed by the inevitable distractions thrown your way during in-class exams.

One explanation for why the busy coffee shop helps is a concept called State-Dependent Memory. Being in the same *state* could allow for easier access to facts and concepts you learned while under similar circumstances. Controversy exists regarding how relevant state-dependent memory is to any given situation, but anyone who has seen *Beerfest* is familiar with the concept: the characters were unable to remember the location of an international beer-drinking tournament... until once again becoming intoxicated.

Digital Technology and Apps

Devices change and improve all the time, so it won't be fruitful to review specific phones, computers or tablets for students, but we think that a few common technologies will be remain relevant for students in the years to come. One is cloud data storage. Many companies provide solid cloud storage platforms for free or minimal cost. We strongly recommend that, if your school doesn't provide this already, you invest in a service that will facilitate safe storage of all your class powerpoints, notes, lectures, and textbooks. Keeping a hard drive backup of these resources is also a good idea.

Along similar lines, as you move further into your career, you will want to find a way to keep track of all those research articles, medical society guidelines, and helpful webpages. Keep these in a single, organized location. Highlights from textbooks, manuals, and other tablet-based media can be saved to note-taking apps as well. It is great to have a direct quote with the article name or page number at your fingertips.

Use Read It Later extensions and phone apps that help you to subscribe to blogs or news feeds of interest. You can simply scroll through and mark numerous articles to read later. Usually, these will also allow you to view in an ad-free format, which by itself makes them worthwhile.

We also recommend using an unsubscribe email app, such as UnrollMe. This free app will monitor your email for any lists that have your email and allow you to easily unsubscribe from them.

There's even "fact-checking" and "fake news" browser extensions these days. There are pros and cons to each of these, but sometimes they can be a useful tool when searching for information that is out of your normal comfort zone. For example, with the International Fact-Checking Network you can view their Signatories list of verified fact-checkers [21]. Sources on this list will usually provide reliable information.

Playing around with some of these technologies now will make it easier to use them well later. Despite how busy you may feel during medical school, it is significantly easier to spend some time experimenting with these now than when you are working 12+ hour shifts as a resident or attending.

Pre-Study Preparation

You may think that after this many pages we would *finally* be ready to study, right? Wrong! Here's the issue with how most of us study: we jump into a study session with plenty of energy and enthusiasm, only to find that we are not yet prepared to use the time well.

This is something we are very familiar with, as we're sure most of you are. What are some ways that we can prepare our bodies to optimize our studying? Some recommend meditation, even a few minutes will be helpful. Others might try breathing exercises, like ten deep/slow breaths before getting started. Still others might respond better to exercise, stretching, or yoga. Whatever helps to keep you happy, healthy, and focused.

If using the ergonomic principles from above, you should also be sitting upright with most or all of your body at 90° angles. Comfort can also translate into longer productive periods of study without need the need to take breaks.

Environmental temperature is an often-overlooked aspect of comfort when studying. Studies of task-specific performance metrics have demonstrated that even a few degrees away from an individual's preferred temperature can greatly impair cognitive performance [22].

One more obvious, yet overlooked, consideration is to declutter your workspace. Especially when limited on space, we may use the same desk or table for studying, reading, eating, and even sleeping from time to time. But to have the most efficient and focused study sessions, it's important to limit distractions [23].

Physical distractions are easy enough to remove. Clear your desk of all non-necessary materials. This doesn't mean simply move it to the far corner of your desk, or even in the desk drawer. You want all non-necessities to be out of eye-sight and out of reach so they are not tempting you. We've heard of some students even putting them in a locked box in another room, though your closet will probably suffice.

Now look down at your desk. Is your phone and/or tablet still sitting there? Is it what you will be completing your work on? If yes to the first and no to the second, put it away. No, you don't need your phone as a timer because your computer has a clock. No, you don't need to look up this or that extra document on your tablet. **Put. It. Away.**

Prevent Phantom Vibration Syndrome, which is just what it sounds like: when your phone is off or on silent and you still think you feel it vibrating [24]. This sensation can even occur when your phone is not in your pocket! FOMO (fear of missing out) is a real issue in medical school, which tempts you to check devices too often and can decrease your motivation to study [25,26]. Here's a brief list of actions that will help to prevent and manage electronic distractions:

1) Put your phone on Do Not Disturb.
2) Take all electronics off WiFi unless specifically needed.
3) If needed, use browser plug-ins like StayFocusd or Timewarp to reduce time on social media and other distractions.
4) Close any browser tabs or apps that you are not actively using to study.
5) Mark on a nearby sheet or whiteboard the number of times you are distracted. Keep this for your record over time to see if distractions are correlated with other aspects of your day or mood (like hunger or fatigue).

New tech, apps, and plug-ins are created all the time, so assuming this book is being read a few years from now, it may be a good idea to search around for the *latest and greatest*. Search "productivity apps" or go on AlternativeTo.net for crowd-sourced recommendations.

We have provided a lot of recommendations, thus far. You may be chomping at the bit to sit down and get to work. But before sliding into your favorite chair, let's place one more finishing touch into the study environment: a houseplant. No, we're not kidding. Interaction with your chlorophyllic roommate may decrease both physiologic and psychologic stress [27], clean the air you breathe, and boost concentration & productivity [28]. Engaging with nature reduces stress and boosts creativity [29]. Although the benefits are likely to be modest, any movement towards the great outdoors can help.

Finally, we are finished with the prep work for our upcoming study sessions. We have discussed how to be more comfortable, more focused, and more efficient. **Experiment with the recommendations that stuck out to you.** You don't need to use every single one. In the next section, we will give an overview of some helpful tips and tricks that will make the process of studying more effective and efficient.

Create a Study Plan

Hopefully, by this stage in your academic career, you have developed proper and adaptable study habits. But few of us were really given guidance on how to study. Most of us learned by trial and error. You have probably heard the saying, *when all you have is a hammer, everything looks like a nail.* Hopefully, this section will give you more tools to get the job done.

Even if you have years of experience developing schedules, to-do lists, and coordinating your responsibilities (school, home, work, personal, etc.) there may still be ways to improve. With such a complex (and often changing) schedule in medical school, it will be essential to thoughtfully prepare your study plan. To get the most out of studying, you'll want to use a few different kinds of resources, which we classify as: **Informative Material, Rehearsal/Recall Material**, and **Practice Material**.

Informative Material consists of in-class lectures, textbooks, Powerpoints, and other forms of primary learning material. This is the focus of most schools which, unfortunately, gives students the impression that this should be their main focus as well. But the preclinical years of medical school are a little different than your previous education. Because so much information is coming so fast, it is essential to establish conditions that allow you to regularly rehearse/recall information and to apply your knowledge with practice questions.

Rehearsal/Recall involves re-reading notes, reviewing flashcards, and setting aside time for open recall (as a monologue or dialogue). For example, you could read your in-class notes on the anatomy of the lower leg, then run through a few flashcards you made, and then go into the anatomy lab and try to identify the structures (by yourself or with a study buddy).

When we say Practice Materials, we really just mean high-quality, board-style practice questions from reputable Qbanks. To name a few, some of the best resources we have seen are UWORLD, Amboss, Kaplan, Osmosis, USMLE-Rx, as well as COMBANK or COMQUEST for osteopathic students. Most question banks worth your time have to be paid for, but there are free options available, like ExamCircle. There are also free, pre-made flashcard decks for Recall/Rehearsal. (Anki flashcard decks are particularly popular among medical students.)

Neglecting any one of the components above is likely to harm your studies; you need to have balance. Focusing too much of your time on Informative Material, for instance, limits your ability to reinforce it with recall and to apply it with practice questions. This is a very common problem we see with the average student and it contributes to the **Illusion of Competence**. As it sounds, this means that we might be tempted to skim through the highlighted sections of our notes and think that we really "know" the material because it sounds familiar. However, when you are presented with the material in a different way (or have to apply it), this kind of superficial understanding just won't cut it.

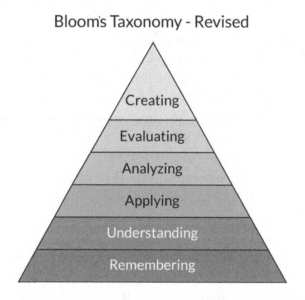

If you were to look at Bloom's Revised Taxonomy, you would notice that *remembering* and *understanding* are at the base of the pyramid. While necessary, they are not sufficient to achieving mastery of a subject. To reach the higher tiers, the bulk of your study time should be dedicated to Recall/Rehearsal and Practice Material.

Using our three types of study material, Informative, Recall/Rehearsal, and Practice, start assembling the first draft of your study plan. Some useful questions to think about here: When will you draw from pre-made vs. self-made materials? How much time will you allocate to each resource you use? Will you need to emphasize different study materials for different disciplines (i.e., anatomy vs. physiology vs. biostats)? The answers to these questions will vary widely across schools, disciplines, time of the year, stress levels, etc. Plus, you'll need to revise your strategy as you go along, so don't feel like you need to have all the answers on day one.

For example, the first few weeks of each new term may be more heavily weighted towards Informative and Rehearsal materials, then as the test approaches, you'll want to incorporate more Practice materials. Evaluate your approach as you trounce one class after another. Being mindful of your thought process and keeping a record of your successes and failures will be helpful. We will cover more on journaling in a later section, but first, we need to finish up our discussion of study techniques.

The **Spacing Effect** is a general educational term for spacing out your study sessions to increase the amount of material you cover and the amount of material you retain. Spaced learning is often contrasted with massed learning. As you can imagine, massed learning tries to get it all done at once, while spaced learning takes advantage of the Spacing Effect. The well-known book, *Make It Stick,* provides strong arguments in favor of spaced learning by showing how and why it yields better test scores and skill development.

The neuroscience behind spaced learning points to physiologic changes in the hippocampus, the region of the brain associated with memory [30]. Though hundreds of neurons are produced each day in the hippocampus [31], their memories seem to be impermanent. Training, such as studying and memory recall, helps these neuronal connections/pathways to persist longer [32]. While there is some debate about the details, it is clear is that spacing out your studies increases long-term retention.

One popular way to space out work and promote productivity is the **Pomodoro technique**. In Italian, *pomodoro* means *tomato,* and the technique's name is a reference to the tomato timer used by Francesco Cirillo who developed it. Traditionally, the Pomodoro technique involved a 25-minute session of work, followed by a 5-minute break. After four repetitions in a row, a longer break is taken: generally 15-30 minutes. Efficiency gurus and educators like to mix and match the amount of time and the break length. Most seem to agree that, after about two hours of work, you need to take a longer break to combat mental fogginess and fatigue.

Though it's not complicated, this is a remarkably powerful technique for getting things done.

> *Note from Greg: When I first heard about the Pomodoro technique, I thought it was... stupid. But, as often happens, I was totally wrong. Now, when faced with the dilemma of starting my work vs. starting a Netflix binge, all I have to do is think of the Pomodoro. "It's just 25 minutes, then I get a break." Once I generate some inertia with the first 25 minutes, I'm ready to roll.*

The POMODORO Technique

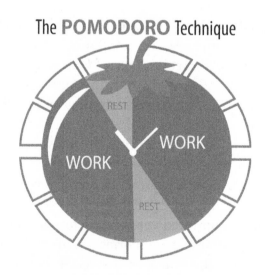

There are also phone apps that can incentivize your studies. Apps like Flora help you to commit to getting a task done with friends, and this commitment is backed up by a monetary pledge. If you don't meet the commitment, then your pledged money will be used to plant a tree. For the purposes of medical school, you could use this kind of app by scheduling a block of time with friends where you aim to review a certain number of lectures or practice questions together. We've given one example, but if you get creative, you'd be amazed by how broadly you can apply this.

The next study strategy that we recommend is **interleaving**. The difference with this strategy, compared to those previously mentioned, is the choice to change up and intermingle the subjects being studied in one sitting. For instance, instead of studying microbiology for two straight hours, you would set a time limit, after which you would study something else. You might do micro for 30 minutes, then anatomy for 30 minutes, then physiology for 30 minutes, and back to micro for the last 30 minutes. Scheduling would depend on your current course load, your strengths & weaknesses, time constraints, etc.

Interleaving is often contrasted with blocking. Where **blocking** has a pattern like AAABBBCCCAAA, **interleaving** has a pattern of ABCACBCBA. Interleaving may benefit a study plan by contrasting the different categories being studied, while blocking emphasizes the similarities within each category of study [33].

So far, we have discussed spacing, interleaving, and the Pomodoro technique to help you develop a schedule that maximizes retention, keeps the content fresh, and keeps you motivated with planned study breaks. Unfortunately, most of us do not have eidetic ("photographic") memory, so multiple repetitions of material will be required. So, our next step is to help you develop a schedule that provides repetition.

When used properly, **Spaced Repetition** is one of the most robust approaches to help our brains remember information over time. Spaced repetition is basically the practice of seeing the information multiple times at increasing intervals. By doing this, you can keep the memory *alive* over a long period of time. The example that immediately comes to mind for medical school is the classic Anki Flashcard deck. This free software has built-in spaced repetition that queues up cards you haven't seen in awhile (and favors the cards you don't know as well). By using flashcards with spaced repetition, we fight the ominous **Forgetting Curve**, which is always lurking in the background to degrade our memories.

Beyond seeing our flashcards at regular intervals, another way we can harness their power is to engage in **Retrieval Practice**, which is a fancy way of saying: *try to come up with the answer on your own, rather than peeking right away.* This principle holds true for any kind of recall activity, not just flashcards.

Evidence supporting the use of Retrieval Practice has been strong in recent years, with the American Psychological Association claiming retrieval to be a key for long-term, durable memories [34]. The strength of formal Retrieval Practice comes from two key factors: 1) it forces the participant to extract and articulate the information from their own memory, rather than relying upon simple word recognition (a pitfall of typical multiple-choice questions); and 2) Retrieval Practice is reinforced with multiple repetitions over time. The graphs shown below demonstrate just how influential these practices can be. There is a significant increase in recall when compared to studying the material once, recalling material once, and even repeated massed study sessions [35].

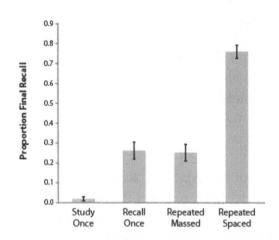

Spaced repetition vs. alternatives, data from Karpicke & Bauernschmidt (2011)

In addition to the improved recall, some studies have shown that the speed of transferring material into long-term memory is significantly greater when using spaced repetition [36]. When done properly, this scheduling technique may be able to save study time and increase recall, which translates into more free time and higher test scores.

We have covered a lot of information in this section. It was meant to be as general as possible to give learners choices to create their own personalized study plan and to avoid the tasks that waste time. Students, unfortunately, get stuck in bad habits like anyone else. We may think that our habits learned in undergrad will be sufficient for medical school, but this is rarely the case.

Some students may be hesitant to try new study strategies in the high-stakes environment of medical school, but if you find yourself struggling to adapt (or simply want to improve), **there's no time like the present to experiment!** Try some of these tactics and record your positive and negative experiences in a journal, or find some other way to objectively monitor them over time. You may also want to check out other well-known educational resources, such as the popular Coursera course, *Learning How to Learn* [37] or the free materials on the Learning Scientists [38] website for more guidance on how to implement these evidence-based techniques.

Now that you have some new tools to help you succeed in scheduling your studies, the next sections will cover how to optimize your study time, point out weaknesses and gaps in your studies, and address these weaknesses.

Efficiency & Time Management

Efficiency and *Productivity* are pretty popular buzzwords these days. People want results, and they want them now! In this section, we will cover some of the better-researched practices for time management. Where evidence may be lacking, we will aim to provide expert opinion. A good place to start our discussion is with an anecdote from the Toyota company.

The *Toyota Production System* was created in the 1940s, but the world did not take notice until the 1970's when Japanese manufacturing began to outperform the U.S. and other global leaders. They used both horizontal and vertical relationships (within their business as well as with external suppliers & distributors), the concept of **Kaizen** (constant improvement), and elimination of waste in all aspects of their business design to become a world leader in car manufacturing [39]. This led to the now-famous "lean" business design commonly used by operations managers.

We can utilize many of these same strategies to enhance our studies. By eliminating waste in as many places as possible, and realizing there is no such thing as perfection, we can learn to strive for continuous improvement or Kaizen.

Focus on Essentials and Take Out the Trash

The **Pareto Principle** [40] (also known as the **80/20 Rule**) is something you will often see in the education, business, and self-help realms. Depending on the source you read, the Pareto principle can be phrased in different ways, but for a medical student, we will describe it this way: for any given topic or lecture, about 20% of the information is need-to-know; by mastering the key 20%, you'll be able to answer about 80% of the questions that come your way. Or you can think of it this way: about 80% of your reward will be gained from 20% of your efforts. The graph below illustrates this point.

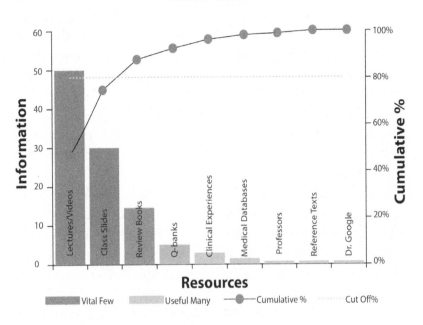

How could we apply the 80/20 rule in medical school? When reading textbooks, you can use the Pareto principle to note or highlight the key points. If you cannot extract the key points from a text, then you don't have enough background to understand the material without the guidance of a teacher. (Or the text is poorly written.) In most textbooks, the key points can be identified by subheadings, bolded words, and summaries at the beginning or end of the chapter. Key points are also reinforced by practice questions provided by the authors. This is the 20% of material that will serve 80% of your needs. Focus on the 20% and you can fill in the blanks later on.

Beyond textbooks, the Pareto principle generally holds true for lectures, labs, problem-based learning, etc. Thankfully, most lectures in medical school are recorded or pre-recorded, allowing the viewer to increase the playback speed to save time. When viewing the lecture at increased playback speed, you will probably miss the minor points, but if the lecturer is doing their job, you will still walk away with the crucial 20%. If anything is unclear, just slow it down or rewind the tape.

When making your study materials (flashcards, outlines, concept maps, etc.), the crucial 20% is the stuff you should plan to have immediately available. The remaining 80% is the filler that you can slowly add on later. When studying medicine, we cannot neglect the details, but if you try to jump into details too quickly, you'll lose sight of the wider framework needed to organize those details (i.e., *lose the forest for the trees*). Hence, most medical schools start with foundational science courses and then build upon the foundations with the details of clinical medicine to produce a durable structure (or web) of knowledge.

So, on a *granular level*, how can you try to build up from the foundations to the intricate details on the roof? **Use this as a guiding example**: when you correctly answer a flashcard question, take the time to ask "What else do I know about this material?" (and then fact-check your responses). If the additional details you came up with are also found in a board review book or another high-yield resource, then you should add those details onto the flashcard. Don't get discouraged if you produce less important facts during this exercise. The whole point is to establish or strengthen connections within your web of knowledge (and to bring in an extra layer of Retrieval Practice to your studies). While this takes more time than quickly rifling through a flashcard deck, we find that it produces deeper learning.

When you're just starting out, focus on mastering the crucial 20% according to the Pareto principle. This helps you to avoid getting bogged down by unimportant details in the 80%, thus eliminating waste in your studies (i.e., taking out the trash). New material comes at you really fast in medical school, so it will take time to learn how to do this well. All we can do is strive for continuous improvement. This is the concept of Kaizen.

Like we discussed before, you ought to mix this kind of active work with regular breaks to maximize efficiency and minimize waste. Now, what should you do while you're on a break? It's up to you, but we would recommend avoiding anything that is mentally taxing or anything that can easily captivate your attention (e.g., social media or television). Some studies show increased attention and focus on study tasks when light physical activity is implemented during break time

[41,42]. Meditation can also reduce stress between study sessions [43].

Of course, you should reward yourself for doing great work, but if there is more studying to get done today, save the unhealthy rewards for the end of the day. Beers with friends or your favorite drama (with a pint of ice cream) can wait until the day is over.

Hopefully, this section on eliminating waste has been helpful. This naturally leads us into a discussion of how to prioritize your time/effort.

Prioritization

"The key is not to prioritize what's on your schedule,
but to schedule your priorities."
Stephen Covey

How do you establish your priorities? Do you focus more on deadlines? On value-added? Steven Covey's Time Management Grid, as described in *The 7 Habits of Highly Effective People*, is a fantastic tool that can help you to prioritize... just about anything. By framing your tasks as urgent vs. non-urgent AND important vs. non-important, it is much easier to identify the tasks that need to be done right now, as opposed to the tasks that can wait. Responding to that email or text may seem urgent and important at the time, but it can probably be put off until more important things are done. Within each box, rank the most critical task within that category at the top of the list. If you're working under a deadline, write down the deadline next to the task.

	Urgent	Not Urgent
Important	**Quadrant I** • Upcoming Deadlines • Exam Dates	**Quadrant II** • Long-term Planning • Recreation • Personal Wellness
Not Important	**Quadrant III** • Interruptions (emails, calls, notifications) • School Activities	**Quadrant IV** • Busy Work • Leisure Activities • Time Wasters

An Adaptation of Covey's Time Management Grid

Category	Task
Important & Urgent: Crisis (keep to a minimum)	Tasks that have made it to this point are often due to procrastination (or last-minute assignments). Avoid filling this section by completing tasks when in the Important/Not Urgent box.
Important/ Not Urgent: High yield	These tasks should generally be completed before anything else. They are the bread and butter of your tasks and lead to the greatest daily yield. Complete these tasks so they do not become Urgent.
Not Important/ Urgent: Interruptions	Emails, phone calls, conversations, and other interruptions can be mitigated by having set times to deal with them. In the *4-Hour Work Week*, Tim Ferris recommends only 1-2 set times per day (example: noon and 8 pm) to complete these tasks so that they are not a constant distraction.
Not Important/ Not Urgent: Time-wasters	Social media, television, and other leisure activities can be used as self-rewards but should never be the focus throughout the day. Even using them as rewards may be detrimental to motivation.

Using this framework, you can easily create your own daily (or weekly) schedule. Or you could adapt an existing schedule that you purchased from your school's bookstore. If you like our style, you can download our template for free at FreeMedEd.org/MedStudent.

A fun way to prioritize is to use a gamified To-do List app, such as Habitica. This *graphically-antiquated* app is a surprisingly good motivator for students. In the simplest terms, it is a medieval-style game in which your character grows as you check off items on your to-do lists. You can customize items by deadline, urgency, and magnitude. You can also join together with other players (classmates) on a quest!

If this point hasn't already become obvious to you, we are in favor of using a system - any effective system - that will help you to keep your thoughts organized and your mind prepared to face the challenges posed by each day. Preparation is paramount. Procrastination is not a strategy for success in medical school. Spending time up-front to set up a proper schedule, flashcard decks, notes, study guides, etc. will serve you well. Not having your stuff ready to go is a recipe for disaster.

By glancing ahead in your textbook, syllabus, or other course guides, you will get a general idea of the type and amount of material you will need to study, which should guide the creation of your study plan. Another strategy is to ask an upperclassman - whose opinion you trust - about how to prepare for each block. By keeping yourself one step ahead, you will have room to adjust your strategies as needed. And, most importantly, you will have gaps in your schedule to relax and recharge.

Goals, Preparation, and Success

Though we often think of mental and physical stress as separate entities, they are not. When you are mentally tired, do you really want to go to the gym? Can you picture going on a 10-mile hike, then coming back to sit at a table and study for 4 hours? Probably not.

In *Peak Performance*, Brad Stulberg and Steve Magness, describe the conclusions of their research into what it takes to excel in all areas of life. Echoing the sage research of psychologists such as Anders Ericsson (author of *Peak*) and Mihaly Csikszentmihalyi (author of *Flow*), both of which will be discussed further in an upcoming section, Stulberg and Magness explain how we can use the growth equation for physical and mental excellence.

The Growth Equation is expressed as, **Stress + Rest = Growth**. This is most often seen in athletes, for whom heavy training intervals are followed by light training to allow for growth and recovery of muscles. This systematic training and improvement schedule has been termed *periodization* in athletics. In order to build our stamina in study habits, we must set up the appropriate mental workout schedule. Let's discuss two tools that can help us organize this schedule.

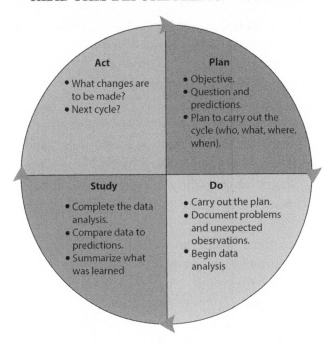

The **Plan-Do-Study-Act method (PDSA)** is a common model for business quality improvement. It is also used in the hospital system and is recommended by the Agency for Healthcare Research and Quality's Health Literacy Universal Precautions Toolkit [44]. This simple wheel is reminiscent of the kaizen philosophy: always improving.

We can utilize this same procedure when examining and changing our study habits. As mentioned in previous sections, our study habits cannot remain static. They are as dynamic as the course materials, instructors, and supplemental resources we encounter. Thinking of study skills as an "I have them or I don't" proposition will be detrimental to your motivation and progress.

The idea behind PDSA is simple: Make a plan. Carry it out. Scrutinize the results to see what works and what doesn't. Make a new plan based on the results. Repeat. Unfortunately, it's easy to say that we will use PDSA to strive for constant improvement, but the execution is just plain difficult. Anyone who gets into medical school is - by definition - intelligent and hard working. We have cultivated many good habits that made us successful, but when our old habits stop working and we encounter failure, it's hard for most of us to adapt. Our instinct is to dig in our heels, thinking that we just need to work harder. But sometimes, that's not the answer. Instead, we need to embrace the change that's needed to succeed in our new surroundings. This is where PDSA shines.

We can supercharge this process by bringing in help, like a study buddy. The book of Proverbs says that, "As iron sharpens iron, so one man sharpens another." This holds true for medical students as well. Surround yourself with a small group of dedicated friends who all have the same vision: successfully educating yourselves in order to take excellent care of your future patients. You'll be amazed by the results.

Okay, that's enough pontificating... What else can we do to set ourselves up for success? PDSA is just a general guideline for the process of quality improvement. Next, you need to drill down on the details of your study goals.

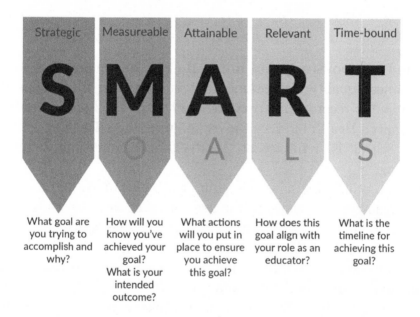

PDSA is particularly powerful when combined with **SMART Goals**, which is a mnemonic that helps you to remember how to craft your goals. You want them to be Specific, Measurable, Attainable, Relevant, and Time-bound.

When crafting our goals, we want to ensure that these goals are truly aligned with our endgame, and not just with our fleeting sense of satisfaction. That may be higher grades in class (not recommended), increased comprehension and synthesis (recommended), or higher board exam scores (unfortunately important). Measuring or completing tasks that do not align with our end-goals will waste precious time.

Let's take a moment to experiment with how PDSA and SMART goals can be used to create a study plan. First, the PDSA method can be used to provide a broad overview of the first steps to making a change to your studies. This could look something like, "I need to pass my course. The teacher recommends the textbook, so I will study exclusively from the textbook."

The Plan is to exclusively use the textbook to review for the course. After you Do this, you Study the results by evaluating your grades after making the change. Then you then Act accordingly: will you continue with this strategy because it worked well? Modify it? Give up on the textbook altogether?

Let's assume that using the textbook worked well. (Just a *hypothetical*.) Afterward, you can start to hone-in on a more specific goal by using the SMART framework. One example would be: "I will increase my dedicated study time by two hours throughout the week, specifically devoting this time to reading the assigned chapters in the textbook. With this change, I expect to see a 5 point increase on the next exam." This describes a Specific increase in our study time and exam grades, Measured in time and points, which is Attainable (we aren't aiming for 20 more hours of work or 20 more points) and Relevant to our broader goals of academic success. Finally, the goal is Time-bound between now and the next exam.

General/vague descriptions of your goal should be avoided. When possible, give yourself hard numbers to compare to. Not setting a completion time is also a common mistake when goal-setting. Think about any vague New Years' resolution you have ever made or heard about; they almost never succeed. Winning strategies tend to use some variant of the PDSA and/or SMART frameworks.

With these goals and tasks now spelled out, you may want to use something like Covey's Time Management Grid (discussed previously) to prioritize your new goals and tasks. The relative priority of goals and tasks should be flexible enough to deal with the changes and challenges inherent to life. It is very easy to assume we have put in X amount of hours to achieve Y grades, or to think that your future self will be more productive with each hour of work than is realistic. This is where a journal can come in handy. You can use it to record your goals, track your progress, and guide your plans for the future.

Efficiency Fights Burnout

One last thing to note before we take a deeper dive into study techniques is the topic of burnout. Unfortunately, the current setup of medical education contributes to burnout among many students. Studies have shown that it is your learning/working environment that contributes the most to burnout, more so than personal characteristics [45-47]. Luckily, there are a few defensive barriers we can try to set up to protect ourselves from a toxic environment.

Framework of Burnout

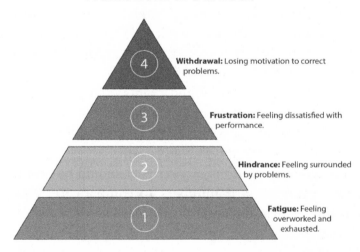

4 **Withdrawal:** Losing motivation to correct problems.

3 **Frustration:** Feeling dissatisfied with performance.

2 **Hindrance:** Feeling surrounded by problems.

1 **Fatigue:** Feeling overworked and exhausted.

Internal defensive barriers to burnout involve regular self-assessment (like mindfulness training). At the end of the day, you have to recognize burnout in yourself. You cannot always rely on others. The four-step Framework of Burnout - fatigue, hindrance, frustration, and withdrawal - helps us to put a label on the common stages of burnout to better understand our feelings. If you *consistently* identify with one or more of these steps, please reach out and seek help.

But who will you reach out to? This is where external defensive barriers come into play. By *external barrier*, we really mean the involvement of other people. Having one or more persons to share your burdens will lighten the load. Ask these people to agree to point out their concerns ahead of time, and agree to a game-plan together. If you don't want to involve someone in your personal life, consider getting a therapist or speaking with a counselor at your school. Resources like TalkSpace can be a great way to get started with therapy. Dr. Dike Drummond (aka The Happy MD) has produced very helpful content for physicians interested in burnout prevention.

This touchy-feely stuff can be off-putting to some personalities, so if this advice doesn't work for you, then figure out another way to combat burnout. Don't assume that you are immune to its effects. As an alternative, you could consider sublimating your frustrations in healthy ways like team sports or passion projects. Avoid destructive means of stress-relief, like alcohol or drugs. (Yes, these are real issues among medical students and physicians [48].)

> *Note from Chase: I can honestly say that I hit ALL of the steps of burnout during my second year of medical school, withdrawing from nearly all my social connections and ignoring solutions to my problems. I was far from the only one.*

Although we will discuss this more in the Work-Life Balance section of this book, learning to become more efficient will do wonders for students on the road to burnout [49]. Of course, many other factors can help too, such as exercise, diet, meditation, etc. One thing you can immediately do to improve your efficiency is to start using a **Checklist**. By externalizing the tasks we need to do onto a checklist, we can drastically reduce anxiety related to forgetfulness and unfinished work. In medicine, particularly the surgical subspecialties, the checklist plays a critical role before, during, and after the operation [50]. By helping us push decision-making *out to the periphery*, checklists minimize human error. This point is hammered home in the popular book, *The Checklist Manifesto*, by Dr. Atul Gawande.

To prove the power of the checklist, the World Health Organization and Harvard Medical School joined forces to put it to the test. The death rate of the surgical practices reviewed was 1.5% before the checklist was applied. After implementation, the death rate dropped to 0.6%, and the post-surgical complication rate was nearly cut in half [51]. This may seem like a fairly small percentage change in mortality, but with nearly 234 million surgeries taking place each year, this simple fix can prevent over one million deaths and tens of millions of post-surgical complications each year [51].

Closing Thoughts on Efficiency & Time Management

Please, please, please, begin to implement these tools **right away**. You will see this advice repeated many times throughout the book. It's great to know about the theory, but until you **put it into practice** you will not actualize any benefits. **Experiment** with different organization and prioritization charts. Put into place behavioral changes that will limit distractions and help with mental decluttering.

If you haven't been taking notes on how you can use some of these strategies, we would recommend that you go back and revisit the sections you found helpful. You don't want this stuff to go in one ear and out the other! Consider copying down any of the helpful quotes, diagrams, tables, etc. After giving it a shot, schedule a time for self-assessment and see where you've been able to make improvements.

Studying for the Big Exam

"Start where you are. Use what you have. Do what you can."
Arthur Ashe

To clarify our aims with this section, we don't want to give you the impression that reading it will automatically enable you to ace the USMLE or graduate at the top of your class. We are not salespeople. We are educators. As such, we strive to be intellectually honest. Any books or programs *guaranteeing* top scores should be viewed with extreme skepticism. Even further, we would argue that - at the end of the day – YOUR EXAM SCORES DON'T REALLY MATTER.

Blasphemy! Some of you may want to throw this book in the trash right now. After all, what is school about, and especially medical school, if not test scores? And that is exactly the mentality that will get you into trouble later on in your career. Fixating on test scores will not really help you to be an excellent physician. What ultimately matters is that you do your best for your patients and your team.

All that being said, you still have to pass your classes and board exams to practice medicine. And you should be motivated to perform at your best. The next section will introduce ways to identify the materials that you need to study for your standardized tests.

How to Choose Efficient/ Effective Study Materials

In the last section, we spent a lot of time discussing how to efficiently schedule your daily activities and to prioritize tasks. Now we are going to focus on how to pick and choose which topics to focus on in your studies, so that your time is spent on learning the high-yield information for your classes and for the boards.

As a medical student in your preclinical years (typically MS 1-2), you will constantly run up against the limits of your knowledge. We have all been there: where we start to accumulate a hodgepodge of medical facts but our understanding of this material isn't mature enough to synthesize into a bigger picture. We listen to lectures and read chapters in textbooks, but what do we actually know? How relevant is one fact over another? How do we learn to anticipate, identify, and focus on the essential points of any given lesson, so that we can use our time wisely?

Traditionally, this has been the job of the lecturer or instructor. But every year, the writers of the board exams will make minor changes to the content and concepts they want to test. With this ever-changing curriculum, you cannot guarantee your instructors have a full grasp on what material will truly be board-relevant. Some instructors are asked to contribute board exam questions, or they may pay attention to announcements that come from NBME/NBOME, but those tend to be the exceptional instructors. Most educators and clinicians are busy people, so they don't have much time to devote to keeping up with the board exams.

Luckily, many **third-party medical education companies** have filled this gap in recent years to help students focus on the content that is most board-relevant. These companies are generally made up of dedicated professionals who follow the trends in examinations and education. Most of their products will require an up-front investment, but their guidance is usually of high-enough quality to warrant spending the money. There are even free online resources that are of similar quality, most of which are stationed on Youtube or podcasts.

Despite concerns that the original intent of the Step 1 score was misappropriated for residency selection [52,53] and a plea from members of the community to change this emphasis on a single metric [54], we were stuck with this monstrosity for quite a long time. Most research correlates higher Step 1 scores with a higher passing rate of future specialty board exams [55]. But really what this means is good test takers are, *go figure*, good at taking tests.

Thankfully, in 2022 the first Step of the USMLE will become a pass-fail test, but many students and educators are concerned that this will simply shift residency program directors' attention to Step 2

CK scores instead [56]. It is certainly a step in the right direction, but who knows what the unintended consequences will be?

Many residency programs are beginning to see the short-sightedness of this logic and are choosing to approach candidates more holistically. You can search for the latest NRMP Program Director Survey for their rankings of importance on a host of factors for resident selection. Some of the top items include interactions with faculty, interpersonal skills, personal statements, and letters of recommendation. Unfortunately, most still rank Step or COMLEX scores as *numero uno*.

So, your score on the board exams matters when applying to residency. No matter how smart you are, you will need to prepare for these exams. You cannot procrastinate when studying for these exams; there's just too much information to know. You will need to work hard, but you should also plan to work smart. One way to organize yourself when planning your studies is to use a conceptual equation from CollegeInfoGeek's book, *10 Steps to Earning Awesome Grades While Studying Less*:

Study equation:
(complexity of course x quantity of material) /
familiarity

The equation expresses a simple concept: you can expect to work harder in classes that are complex, that cover a lot of material, and that you are unfamiliar with. Because this is medicine, we can assume the material will be complex and abundant. So, for most medical students, you can expect to allocate the bulk of your study efforts on the material that you are least familiar with.

As an example, biochemistry usually ranks low in familiarity and high in complexity. In your preclinical courses, there will be a significant amount of biochemistry to study, but a relatively small fraction of that material will be critical for the boards and wards. Make sure you pay close attention to topics like oxyhemoglobin dynamics and acid-base balance, but the minutiae of the Krebs cycle are not worth committing to memory for the long term. So, even though biochemistry will require considerable effort, it is not as high-yield as subjects like anatomy or pharmacology.

You should also consider the 80/20 Rule when approaching any given subject: you can learn most of what you need to know in a relatively short amount of time, but if you try to squeeze in every last detail, there will be diminishing returns for your extra effort. After all, there are only 24 hours at your disposal each day, so you will need to prioritize.

The next step is to understand your strengths and weaknesses. Once we have laid down the foundation for our house of knowledge, we can start to fill in the important structural gaps and to connect different areas of the house to transform it from a hollow shell into a cohesive unit. Medical board exams like to test your critical thinking skills by posing questions that require you to synthesize information across disciplines while applying your understanding to a unique clinical scenario. If you have gaping holes in your house of knowledge, it will be very challenging to answer these kinds of complex questions. So, one of your goals during your pre-clinical courses needs to be identifying and filling in your knowledge deficits.

Knowledge

		Knowns	Unknowns
Metaknowledge	known	known Knowns	known Unknowns
	unknown	unknown Knowns	unknown Unknowns

To organize your approach to identifying knowledge deficits, you could use the chart above, which is known as the Johari Window. Though commonly misattributed to a speech given by Donald Rumsfeld (former US Secretary of Defense), this organizational schema was actually created by two psychologists studying group dynamics in the 1950s. This tool could be helpful to organize your knowledge gaps into high vs. low priority.

For example, by definition, we cannot have knowledge in the Unknown Unknowns category. We have to be introduced to it first, then we can then use other resources to help classify it into high vs. low priority. The way this would work in medical school is to be introduced to a topic in your classes, then to classify it as high vs. low priority based on what you see in third party review materials.

In contrast, there are the Known Knowns which we already know very well. From previous exposure and study, we have already mastered this content, so we never miss these questions on an exam. While it's great to feel this sense of mastery, it's still important to stay humble because the Forgetting Curve is always at work!

Unknown Knowns might represent material that you unassumingly knew from past experiences, such as when you broke your arm as a child. While being treated by a doctor, you were passively absorbing a lot of information from the medical environment. As a result, you might have more knowledge and experience than you initially thought regarding fractures, the imaging required, how to fit a cast, etc. before you sit down to study. This is often the kind of material that your brain just seems to resonate with, so there is no need to apply great effort when learning these topics. Simply review them and move on.

Known Unknowns are probably best depicted by quiz/test questions that we have gotten wrong. The question identified a clear knowledge gap, so we would expect to benefit from focusing our efforts here. You ought to take notes or create flashcards for this type of material. Plan to review it at regular intervals to reap the rewards of spaced repetition. If you are using programs that have built-in spaced repetition, like Anki, they will usually identify your weak points and handle the scheduling of long-term review for you. Additionally, if you use an online question bank for personal learning/quizzing, it will usually provide a breakdown of correct vs. incorrect questions by discipline. Part 2 of this book has a segment that will provide you with the relative importance of each discipline for the board exams.

Monitoring Study Habits and Improvements

Thus far, we have found the best material to study, identified knowledge gaps, and have our SMART Goals selected. But we need to make sure we are able to stay on the right track. How can we stay motivated?

There are two basic forms of motivation: intrinsic motivation and extrinsic motivation. Most employers will focus on providing extrinsic motivators for their employees, like wages, holiday bonuses, benefits, etc. in order to boost worker productivity and morale. However, behavioral economists and those who study business management know that extrinsic motivation can only get you so far.

Intrinsic motivators, on the other hand, shape our interests and desires, without the expectation of external reward. Recent studies show a stronger correlation between academic success and intrinsic motivation than extrinsic motivation [57]. But medical students are already intrinsically motivated and highly successful people. How then could medical students boost their own intrinsic motivation to an even higher level? Students in higher education tend to experience greater motivation from verbal rewards than tangible rewards [58]. And some studies even show that tangible extrinsic rewards can be detrimental to intrinsic motivation [59]. So, instead of buying yourself a treat for completing the task, perhaps a bit of positive self-affirmation or a pep talk from a good friend would be better ways to stay motivated?

Regardless of how you try to hack your own motivation, it will require some trial and error. For example, if you find that creating concept maps provides more satisfaction than typing out a study guide, then you should try to use the former strategy as much as possible. Obviously, you'll need to have multiple study strategies depending on the subject - different tasks will require different tools - so try to find a few new strategies throughout this book that you like to use. It may be easier to do the burdensome (less intrinsically motivating) tasks in the morning when you are fresh, and you can save the refreshing (more intrinsically motivating) tasks for when you're running out of steam.

In *The Power of Habit*, Pulitzer Prize-winning reporter, Charles Duhigg argues that all habits - including study habits - follow the same basic loop, from Cue to Routine to Reward. The Habit Loop eventually forms a Craving, which is an anticipation of the reward to come. These cravings can lead to pleasurable dopamine spikes, just from thinking about the reward to come. This model is easily applied to addiction, but also describes our habits in everyday life.

Duhigg further describes how Keystone Habits are mutable activities or traits that can spark a change in other areas of life. Probably the most important one to cultivate is your *willpower*. Willpower really can be thought of as a habit like any other. Stress can eat away at your willpower throughout the day. However, willpower can also be strengthened, like a muscle, by steadily increasing the number of tasks you resolve each day. By accumulating "small wins" day-in and day-out, many people will experience a greater sense of agency and competence, thus building up willpower. In medical school, this could be achieved by breaking down your reading assignments or video lectures into smaller bits, like 1-2 page sub-sections of a textbook or 15-20 minutes of a 90-minute lecture. Then you could incorporate interleaving by switching between small tasks during the workday to keep yourself engaged with the material.

Of course, we can't discuss good habits and leave out the bad. According to Duhigg, we can never truly eliminate bad habits. However, we can redirect the Habit Loop by keeping the Reward and altering the Routine. When you receive the Cue, whether it be a marketing ad, a computer pop-up, or an internal sensation, try to identify a healthier alternative Routine to get the same Reward.

The example he uses is the Habit Loop for smoking. The Cue could be your morning coffee. The Reward is the neurochemical rush that smoking offers. Instead of falling into the same old Routine, when the Cue hits your senses, try to focus your energy into performing 20 push-ups rather than lighting up. It is amazing to realize that different Routines can still produce the same Reward (i.e., increased dopamine). By re-directing our Routine, we can turn a bad habit into a good Habit Loop. With a little bit of self-reflection, we could certainly use this internally-focused schema to form better habits around studying.

Alternatively, much of the current literature on Habit-based Intervention focuses on making environmental (external) changes. It is much easier, after all, to avoid the ice cream and potato chips isles in the grocery store than it is to refrain from eating them when they are already in your kitchen. By intentionally shaping your environment ahead of time, you can nudge your future self into better habits. This is a place where accountability partners can make a difference too. By planning to grocery shop together on a designated day of the week, you can encourage each other to steer clear of the junk isles.

The parallels to studying are numerous. One example that immediately comes to mind is the bad Habit Loop related to cell phones. The Cue is a buzz or alert sound; the Routine is to reflexively pull out your phone and check the message; the Reward is the little dopamine hit provided by instantly gratifying your curiosity. But then you delve into other updates, scroll across your social media feeds, or do a few searches. And by the time you look up, you've lost a few minutes of life and have derailed your study progress. We are all guilty of this. So, a simple fix is to set up your study environment with your phone on silent (ideally in another room). Or you could uninstall your social media apps. Or find some other workaround. The end goal of studying is intellectual growth and achievement, not instant gratification.

> *Note from Greg: While I was writing this section, my phone kept buzzing in my pocket and I felt myself straining to not check it. The irony was not lost on me.*

So, how can you incorporate good habits into the classroom? The 2014 book, *Make it Stick*, is one of the great modern summations of educational literature. Among other things, this book advocates for teachers and learners to take advantage of the Testing Effect (pre- and post-testing) and the Practice Effect (spaced retrieval) with frequent and smaller testing sessions incorporated into every single lecture or activity. The pre-test primes the learner to important facts to come. The post-test points out weak spots in the student's understanding and guides their future studies. Spaced retrieval helps to fight against the Forgetting Curve.

If your school does not already incorporate these methods by default, then make sure to test yourself to boost your learning. At the end of each lecture, close your notes and try to recall (or even write down) as many of the important subjects and terms as you can. This can take as little as 30 seconds and harnesses the power of immediate Retrieval Practice, which will be discussed in later sections of this book. After recalling what you remember, scan through the lecture slides and highlight or otherwise note any important areas that you missed. If you have a study partner in class, class breaks are the perfect time to quickly quiz each other. Seeing what someone else found memorable can be quite valuable because you can use each others' understanding to gain new insight into the material. In particular, you should be curious about how they linked some of the key ideas and facts together.

Next, when you exit the classroom, you'll need to have a game plan for how you will allocate your time in self-study. After all, if we're using the majority of home study time simply to create study materials, but ultimately spend little time reviewing those materials, then we've missed the boat. During a workday, we need to ensure that we can appropriately allocate our time-spent on any given task. To learn how to effectively allocate time, we can glean some wisdom from the business world.

Now, this next series of questions may seem random, but we promise that it's relevant: How does your local ice cream shop set their prices? Are you charged a different price for a scoop of *vanilla* compared to a scoop of *double-chocolate fudge brownie*? Probably not. But the managers of any business must know the cost of each product or service. They do this by breaking down the numbers to look at production cost vs. returns for each of their products and then making comparisons between products. How else would you know if *pumpkin spice* is becoming an expensive sinkhole while *strawberry shortcake* has made 80% of the profits for this month?

If pumpkin spice isn't profitable, then the manager will stop stocking it in the freezers, opting for more strawberry shortcake instead. This is known as **activity-based costing** (ABC). Obviously, this is a very valuable practice to businesses and individuals, which is why any bank or credit union will provide you with an account statement each month. Online banks or budgeting apps like Mint also provide you with spending category breakdowns, including line items like gas, groceries, restaurants, utilities, etc. so you can monitor where your money is going each month. Hopefully, it's not all going to impulse buys and beer.

As a medical student, you could use the principles of ABC to optimize your study efforts. For example, if you were to commit to using a time-tracking app like Toggl for a week, you could get a baseline breakdown of how you spend each day. Perhaps you find that cooking your meals each day is taking up 2 hours of time when you thought it only took 30 minutes. If this is the case, you could consider doing meal preparation, dedicating 3-4 hours of time on the weekend to prep all your meals for the week. This would save you 10-11 hours of time each week, which you could redirect elsewhere.

How could this apply to studying? When studying, you also have "line items" like materials creation, self-review and rehearsal, and group study. If you want, you could break these down even further. The figures below provide an example of time tracking for a student, divided into "In School" and "Out of School" activities.

The relative utility of each activity depends on personal preference and effectiveness. Further, these categories will change depending on the timing of your exams. For example, creating new study materials can and will take a considerable amount of time. This is time well-spent early in the semester because it forces you to dig in deep to understand the material. However, as your tests approach, you will naturally switch into review mode. Similarly, self-assessment with question banks is likely to be less helpful at the beginning of the semester but will increase in importance later on. Regardless of how your time is spent initially, keeping a record of your time and correlating it with your exam performance (and overall wellbeing) will be helpful to guide your future decisions.

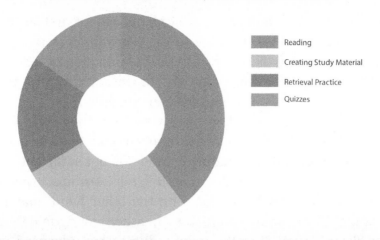

	Prep	Health & Wellness	Study & Review	Leisure	Quizzes	Daily/ Weekly Total
In School	30%	10%	38%	2%	20%	100%
Outside of School	20%	15%	50%	5%	10%	100%

Assessing and Improving your Learning Abilities

Many students never stop to *really* consider how they learn best or to consider how the best learning method will change, based on the task at hand. Most of us just pick up learning habits through years of trial and error. We fumble along until we make it to the next stage, but if we take the time to internalize the mental constructs and processes that support learning, there's a lot of improvement to be had.

It is a common misconception among students that learning styles - specifically the Visual - Auditory - Reading - Kinesthetic (VARK) styles - are a critically important consideration when planning their studies. Teaching to an individual's preferred learning style does not necessarily yield better academic results [60].

By emphasizing one component (audio, video, reading, etc) over the others, you limit the student's routes of exposure to the material. Further, different subjects will plainly require different media to get the point across. For example, most students cannot first learn about heart murmurs from just listening to the murmur. Instead, they will need to simultaneously be exposed to the combination of the murmur audio, the anatomic listening point, and the visual waveform to really pick up on the subtle distinctions between murmurs.

A learner who claims not to need visual teaching tools will still need to SEE the brachial plexus to really understand its anatomy. Language, for auditory and reading learners, is not sufficient by itself to explain these kinds of complex anatomic relationships, especially to first-time learners. A neurosurgeon, on the other hand, may have a good enough idea of what's going on when her colleague describes a brachial plexus lesion over the phone, due to her advanced mental representations of the anatomy. But a first-year medical student will not.

Regardless of your preference, you will likely benefit from using ALL of the "learning styles" in conjunction. By using multiple types of media to engage with a topic, we create a powerful learning environment. Like dual-coding, using multiple sensory stimuli encodes information in different manners in the brain. Even rehearsing out loud or repeating material silently to yourself may increase long-term retention [61]. This is thought to be due to the **Production Effect**, where saying material out loud makes it more distinct in the mind and easier to recall later on. Now you have multiple neuronal circuits to call upon when trying to retrieve a particular bit of information. Dual-coding is an important topic for long-term memory and will be brought up again in the Accelerated Learning sections.

Deliberate Practice

"There are no traffic jams on the extra mile."
Zig Ziglar

If you're looking for a rock-solid approach to improve your studies (or any other skill for that matter), look no further than **Deliberate**

Practice (DP). DP, originally described by Dr. Anders Ericsson, has become more popular in recent years because it is a remarkably powerful tool for self-improvement. Dr. Ericsson has summed up his several decades of work in his most recent blockbuster, *Peak.*

Malcolm Gladwell popularized a misinterpretation of Ericsson's work in his book, *Outliers,* which you may have heard of as the "10,000 Hour Rule" for mastery. Despite this setback, Ericsson's work has established a step-by-step manual for mastery of nearly any subject or skill. If you're going to spend thousands of hours to become a doctor, you might as well plan to do it right the first time by getting into the habit of DP while studying.

Deliberate practice, Ericsson claims, is the best method of learning and has virtually no limitations. By repeatedly pushing yourself *just* past your comfort level, but not pushing to the point of burnout, you can steadily master anything. With an organized plan and a dedicated trainee, results will follow. Above all, Ericsson stresses the point that practice is meant to be effective, not fun.

Similar to the idea of the Growth Equation, Ericsson points out that we cannot improve ourselves if we remain in homeostasis. The body and mind must be challenged and put under stress to grow. For instance, some research suggests there is growth in the hippocampus (a region associated with memory formation) in those who regularly challenge their memory [62]. Focal cortical thickening has also been demonstrated with cognitive training [63]. So, in theory at least, when students implement sufficiently stressful study regimens, they are literally reshaping their brain to adapt to the stress. But when we stick to the same old, stress-free routine we never leave the bubble of homeostasis, which means no growth.

Deliberate Practice also emphasizes shaping your own potential with a clear mental representation of the finish line. Articulating a specific goal (like a SMART goal), planning how to get there, and then putting in the hard work will lead you down the path to mastery. Then, you need to record your results and tinker with your approach to continue improving. DP requires you to ruthlessly identify your weaknesses and figure out a way to fix them.

But what if we don't know how to get to that end goal, despite setting SMART goals and revising them regularly? In every stage of knowledge acquisition, there will be roadblocks. This is traditionally where a **teacher or mentor** can assist with their years of accumulated experience/wisdom. In medical school, you'll have instructors of all stripes. Some instructors will be masters of their craft. Others may have no idea how to adequately convey their knowledge down to a medical student level. Here are a few tips we summarized from *Peak* to help you find a good mentor:

1) Find someone who knows the subject very well. For medical education, this could be a clinician who is an expert in their field or possibly an educator who helps to write questions for the board exams. You can also hire medical tutors and others to fill this role if the options from your school do not fit your needs. Proper mentors will probably have published in their field or have awards related to their field.

2) Make sure the mentor provides **frequent and immediate feedback**. Feedback is the cornerstone of deliberate practice. You need to know about your mistakes right away in order to correct them. This is echoed in *Make It Stick* as well.

3) Ignore online rankings. They are highly subjective and prone to biased responses (both bad and good ones). For the most part, it's best to judge a colleague based on your personal interactions with them, rather than relying on hearsay. Free consults, especially for independent contractors, can help with the process of choosing a mentor but are not always available.

4) Make sure you understand your main goals well enough to articulate them to your mentor. Clearly communicate the direction you want to go, so your mentor doesn't misinterpret the endgame. And never let a mentor talk you into something that you're not 100% on-board with. Nobody is perfect and sometimes a mentor will (unwittingly) give you bad advice.

Whether you are studying independently, in a group, or with a mentor, the following cycle describes the progress of DP: **try, fail, explore, try again**. Note the similarity between deliberate practice and the PDSA model (plan, do, study, act). Time after time, effortful practice towards a goal has been shown to be *the* necessary factor for mastery, not natural talent.

Closing Thoughts on Study & Review

This has been a wide-ranging section. There is a lot of overlap in the purpose and design of many of the tools and strategies we covered. There was also some overlap with the previous section, Efficiency and Time Management. Let's sum up the key points.

1) Although we must focus on learning for the board exams, do not let worrying about scores cloud your true academic/career path.

2) Use the PDSA Method and set SMART goals to formulate short-term and long-term plans.

3) Use the Pareto (80/20) Principle, Time Management Grid, and other tools to prioritize your efforts.

4) If you're having trouble motivating yourself to work, try using the Pomodoro Technique to get some traction.

5) Once you've started studying, use Blocking, Interleaving, and Spaced Repetition to make the most out of your time.

6) Avoid Burnout and the Illusion of Competence by recording your experiences in a journal and by performing regular self-assessments.

7) Deliberate Practice. Period.

There is no such thing as perfect. Remember the concept of kaizen, the constant struggle for self-improvement. We all have a long road ahead of us. Now, equipped with new tools and tactics for the job, you WILL be better prepared for the road ahead. The next sections will be brief overviews of the science behind collaboration and Study Groups, as well as Optimizing your Work-Life Balance.

Study Groups

Pre-Test: On a scale of 1-7 (1 = never and 7 = always) rate these questions.

#	Question/Statement	SCORE
1	I pick groups/teams based on ability and make sure we have a shared vision.	/
2	I have a goal in mind and a plan to get there for group projects and study groups.	/
3	I assess what parts of group projects I think work and those that do not.	/
4	I have plans to combat inefficient group times, conflicts and power struggles.	/
	TOTAL	/28

Study groups are a tricky thing, no matter what academic setting you're in. In fact, many professional tutors will advise you to avoid them. On the other hand, collaboration is often praised as a means to produce better results with a diversity of opinions. However, it is not always clear how to get a group to work well.

Teams are increasingly being emphasized in clinical medicine. From the hospital floor to the operating room, learning to work effectively with your team is a necessary skill for any doctor. Miscommunications not only strain the work environment but may also cause harm to patients [64].

In this section, we will explore how, when, and why study groups can be beneficial. There are some very common mistakes made within these social arrangements, and avoiding them from the get-go will help to increase your chances for success.

Member Selection

"You are the average of the five people
you spend the most time with."
Jim Rohn

There are many instances where you may not be able to choose your team members, like with an in-class project or when working on the hospital floor. However, when you pick your study groups outside of class, there are some general rules you may want to follow to optimize your group's ability to function.

In entrepreneurial and business circles, the term *mastermind* is commonly used to depict a group of individuals who gather together to share ideas, experiences, and plans so that they may learn from one another. In fact, some of these groups require huge down-payments to join, sometimes $50,000 or more! If they can command that price tag, they must be doing something right. Below are tips for running a group, fashioned after the mastermind model:

Respect: One highly recommended trait is to pick individuals whose ideas or knowledge you respect. You probably do not want members who regularly speak before fact-checking. This Misinformation Effect [65] can negatively bias your recall in the future, which will cost you points on the test, time to re-learn the material, and (worst-case) produce an error on the wards. If you find yourself in this kind of situation, you should either try to remedy it or consider leaving. If you cannot respect what they say, then why lock yourself into a group contract? Be on the lookout for classmates whose abilities you admire.

Choose those who give you a competitive edge: We all have weaknesses. Finding members whose strengths can fill in your weaknesses is a great way to increase the group's success. The same goes for every other member of the group (where your strengths buttress their weaknesses), such that each person contributes to and benefits from the group synergy.

Assess for diversity and antagonism: Diversity in group settings is a double-edged sword. On one hand, it can generate more group creativity and productivity. However, too much diversity may lead to frustration, personality clashes, arguments, and sabotage. Creating a safe group environment to learn is critical.

Equality: Make sure to pick members who will put in the work but not steal the stage. Too much or too little effort from one individual can make the rest of the group feel underappreciated or overwhelmed. At the end of the day, you're all going to be doctors, so you all need to master the material. Having group members who dominate the conversation or who do not come prepared generates feelings of resentment.

Shared Vision: Not everyone joins a study group for the same reasons. Make sure that your group members are in agreement about their goals and plan. Some students have high aspirations while others are aiming to stay in the middle of the pack. If you're in the former category, then you should surround yourself with kindred spirits. You can't be a rockstar if your bandmates are only willing to play in the garage.

*To help put together a group, you can find a copy of the Study Group Assessment in the Appendix.

Study groups are no easy task. Whether they are purely transactional academic relationships, or you are trying to build your "tribe," forming an effective team is a tough but worthwhile endeavor. Remember, this is a group with whom you should be able to spend a lot of time, during which you will open up and share your thought processes.

Each person needs to appreciate that all the other **members are**

learning the material in real-time. Beyond having the chance to air out your own thoughts, creating a safe space to grow academically is a refreshing experience, as each learner can absorb how the others reached their conclusions, made mistakes, and corrected course. In a way, this can be like the feedback needed for Deliberate Practice. However, it requires that the members trust each other enough to open up and become slightly vulnerable.

With a little effort (and luck), team members may become more than *study buddies*. They can be your social supports during the trying times ahead. Strong social support systems positively correlate with resilience and are thought to protect against burnout [66-69]. Your study buddies may even become your best friends and help you to expand your professional network in the future.

If you're just starting out and unsure about the group, you may even consider taking surveys like the Team Climate Inventory to estimate how well your group will work together. This would likely be overkill, but it might just help you gain some insight about your team's potential [70], while the Group Environment Questionnaire can help gauge group cohesion [71]. Other team-based assessments exist as well. The usefulness of any given assessment will depend upon the type of team involved, the setting, the size, and the group's intentions.

Regardless of what you may personally think about group work, medicine has shifted away from the "lone wolf" physician in recent years, instead opting for healthcare *teams* that can provide better holistic care for the patient. You won't always have your choice of team members, but don't forget that there are resources available to help you do the best with what you have.

Making a Game Plan for the Team

Now that your study team has assembled, what's next? Hopefully, your group has a game plan or ground-rules for moving forward together. Just like in any relationship, it's best if everyone in the group acknowledges the expectations upfront. Here are some important considerations for any study group:

Environment: In this technology-enabled world, we have so many more options than in years past. Though one of the most common places for a group to study is still a Library Study Room, we can just as easily host online meetings on Skype, Zoom, Google Hangouts, etc. The Share Screen function can be just as useful as a whiteboard. If you choose to do virtual meetings, plan to account for video time lags and set rules to limit group members from speaking over each other.

Format: Is this going to be a group discussion, individual lecture, a combination, or some other format? Will there be Q&A? What amount of time is allotted for each part?

Clear Agenda: Not only does the format need to be clear, but the actual topics to be discussed during each meeting should be clear. This can allow team members to prepare materials and questions ahead of time. The more prepared each member is, the more productive the meeting will be.

Task Division: One major advantage of a successful study group is that they can save time for each member. By dividing up the time-intensive work of breaking down each chapter or lecture into its essential components, each member only needs to complete a fraction of the work on their own.

Note from Greg: "During my pre-clinical years, I

studied nearly every lecture with a group of 5-6 other people. The group came together organically in the first week of school and we stuck together all the way through. As an alternative to dividing up the work, we decided to grind through each lecture as a group in a study room on campus, playing the video recording on a shared screen. While we all steadily digested the lecture, one person would write up its study guide (also on a shared screen). After each PowerPoint slide, we would pause the video and group members would take a stab at how to best phrase each line of the study guide. This allowed each person to be heard, to be challenged, and to grow. It was a fantastic success! This approach to group study allowed each of us to do the hard work of digesting the material ourselves, but in a dynamic (mostly fun) group setting."

There are plenty of apps available that can help any group (yes, even a study group) stay organized and keep its members on-task. One popular app, Trello, is based on the Kanban Card design that was created by Toyota in the 1940s. Toyota created physical cards with tasks, and the person holding the card was expected to complete the task. Modern variations of the Kanban Card system allow all members of a team to visualize the tasks at hand. Integration between apps, such as Trello and Slack, allows members to tag each other with tasks, work in subgroups, and check off the completed tasks for all to see.

If these tools are new to you, there is a bit of a learning curve but their overall utility outweighs the upfront time costs. Plus, you can use them for any kind of group work, not just for school. We intend to use them as a regular part of our medical practice.

If the advice above seems *too structured*, you can always try to wing it. However, you may find the rewards of an off-the-cuff study group to be underwhelming. Study groups tend to move slower than individuals, so you want to make sure the time spent was worth your while. Always keep in mind that time is your most valuable resource.

Improving Collaborative Skills

In *Collaborative Intelligence,* Dr. Dawna Markova and Angie McArthur describe the different types of Mind Patterns that people use to communicate. Though the categorical similarities to learning styles are obvious, the authors state this is not meant to be mistaken for a learning style or personality trait. The three overarching types of Mind Patterns are Visual, Kinesthetic, and Audio.

Our collaborative intelligence (CQ) is said to be made up of all three of these, and the order of strength is what separates us into one of six groups: VAK, VKA, KAV, KVA, AVK, and AKV. None of these groups are "better" or "worse" than the others, but developing the skill to move seamlessly from one pattern to the next is worth exploring. You can identify your CQ Mind Pattern with their quiz at CQthebook.com/quiz.

Identifying your own Mind Pattern should be relatively easy, as we all have preferences and naturally find certain content exciting vs. dull. The difficult part is to identify what pattern you attribute to others in your group. But by being aware of what material keeps certain members engaged while others drift off you could intuitively predict their Mind Patterns. Or you could even do the CQ Mind Pattern assessment as a team. Test the waters. You can find a link to the CQ Checklist among our references [72].

When you have an idea of the overall CQ of the group, you can try to arrange group study to maximally engage each member. Those who seem stuck in their head when someone is speaking but are very active when sketching out diagrams or outlines may have a kinesthetic- or visual-dominant pattern. Have this person work on your study guides, mind maps, and outlines. Those that are confidently verbose may be high in audio but shy away from the visuals. Have this person talk things out with the group. Ask the group for feedback about what has worked or hasn't worked in the past.

Another book that we found helpful when considering group study was Paul Skinner's, *Collaborative Advantage.* Skinner argues that fighting for Competitive Advantage (trying to outperform one another) is a sub-optimal strategy when colleagues and students are trying to work together. The world is becoming increasingly complex, so there simply is no way for an individual to know everything. By focusing on a common goal or purpose, we can foster innovation and create more resilience through collaboration. Students should leverage each other's strengths in order to progress further and faster than one would independently.

Though Skinner's book focuses on business and leadership collaboration, similar conclusions have been found in medicine. A Cochrane Review found that greater interprofessional collaboration leads to better healthcare outcomes [73], and the American Heart Association found that collaborative medication reviews also provide positive outcomes [74]. Becoming a skilled collaborator takes time, but it is a powerful tool and well worth the effort.

When it's Time to Change Things Up

Even with a proper member selection process and study strategy, your first few meetings may seem to go sideways rather quickly. All is not lost. Here are a few considerations that may prove useful.

Identify the issues at hand and make a plan to correct them. Solicit help and advice from other members or mentors. When members are made part of the decision-making process, they are more likely to accept and adhere to the decisions made. For some changes, it may be best to first ask members individually to take the overall pulse of the group. Then, synthesize the final decision in a group discussion.

If possible, try to quantitatively assess and monitor changes to ensure they accomplish the desired effects. If there are issues with adhering to timelines, use a stopwatch. If there are concerns with dominant personalities taking charge of a meeting, utilize the concept of the "speaking stick" where only the person in possession of said stick may speak. When stuck, there are plenty of blogs and vlogs on business, psychology, sociology, etc. that may present helpful tips.

One easily overlooked idea in group settings, as well as in organizational structure in general, is that of Job Crafting. This term, researched and coined by Dr. Amy Wrzesniewski, basically formalizes the idea that putting people into positions that are better-suited to their skills and interests will produce superior outcomes [75,76].

Helping teammates become committed to their work will ultimately benefit the entire team. This can be a difficult topic in academic environments, especially one as competitive as medicine. We are expected to know everything, do everything, and be good at everything. This is unrealistic of course, so the high bar and undefined benchmarks can add unnecessary stress in any study group where members are expected to perform week-in and week-out.

When possible, limit burdens and be flexible by allowing members to interact organically, so each person can find their niche within the group. Some situations may feel unequal, where one group member seems to take on an unfair amount of responsibility. But if the group has established a groove that works, why rock the boat? If you try to force equal responsibilities on everyone, the group may actually suffer because you failed to account for the effect of specialization. This is a concept well-known to traditional economists.

That being said, not everyone will be aware of their personal strengths. The Center for Positive Organizations through the University of Michigan, of which Dr. Wrzesniewski is a research member, offers free online tools and workshops at JobCrafting.com. If more ideas are needed, a Wiki search of Group Development will quickly convince you that there is a plethora of possibilities that can improve your study group's dynamic. Pick one and try it out. And don't be afraid to change things up.

Optimizing Work, Life, and Work-life Balance

Pre-Test: On a scale of 1-7 (1 = never and 7 = always) rate these questions.

#	Question/Statement	SCORE
1	I understand my perceptions and how they may differ from the perceptions of others.	/7
2	I look at stressful situations as a challenge to overcome.	/7
3	I know how to implement emotional intelligence in public and private events.	/7
4	I have a physical health plan and monitor it regularly.	/7
5	I have a spiritual health plan and monitor it regularly.	/7
6	I understand the importance of developing leadership skills and have a plan to develop as a leader in my community.	/7
7	I understand there are different ethical frameworks and will try to understand others' views to solve problems.	/7
8	I know the types of journaling habits allotted to me and have a plan to use them.	/7
	TOTAL	/56

Note from Chase: "I find it frustrating and curious that - despite working on dozens of college campuses - I have encountered little discussion about how students pursing advanced degrees are supposed to balance their personal and professional responsibilities. There is insufficient emphasis in higher education on understanding personal cognitive psychology for learners and educators. There is also minimal attention paid to the importance of self-

awareness and self-care."

In this section, we will try to sum up what we think about some of the great insights provided by modern psychological science. We will specifically focus on the topics relevant to medical students. Some of these insights are relatively new, so the research may still be in flux by the time you are reading this.

We will cover topics like stress, grit, burnout, and how to take care of your mind and body. Even though it may stray away from the more academic themes of previous sections, we can confidently say that the content will be important to your academic and professional life.

Your mental and physical health will influence your efficiency, productivity, grades/evaluations, and your interactions with colleagues. Your self-awareness will determine your ability to plan for the future, to stick to changes, and to grow. At the end of the chapter, we have a list of videos and books that we recommend you check out.

Perception & Mindset

"Enthusiasm is common. Endurance is rare."
Angela Duckworth

There is something about persistence that has always confounded us. From athletes to business executives to your average Joe, most will say that persistence is a necessary part of the success equation. But how much of the equation is it? Dr. Angela Duckworth's book, *Grit*, tries to answer this question. Though a basic level of Talent, she argues, is required to gain a Skill, **it is Effort that trumps everything else**. She provides two conceptual equations based on her years of research:

Talent x Effort = Skill and
Skill x Effort = Achievement
Rearranged: **Talent x Effort^2 = Achievement**

As a medical student (or an applicant), you have already proven you have the Talent (or knack) for biomedical science. Next, you need to put in the consistent Effort required to earn that MD or DO. But not all effort is the same. The kind of effort we should all be striving for is best described as Deliberate Practice, which we discussed earlier. Your talent combined with Deliberate Practice WILL result in wonderful achievements.

Duckworth asserts that there are 4 Paragons of Grit: Interest, Practice, Purpose, and Hope. Luckily for us, she also believes Grit to be a plastic (or modifiable) trait. We can alter our "grittiness" through practice and incremental achievements. Like we saw with *The Power of Habit*, small and continuous movement in the right direction can keep us motivated and working towards our ultimate goals, forming a positive feedback cycle of achievement.

Hopefully, you found this segment on Achievement and Grit to be encouraging. Now, we recommend that you take the Grit Scale if you wish to know more about yourself. You could even take it at regular intervals to track the progression of your grit over time. The scale can be found at Dr. Duckworth's website listed in our references [77].

As you utilize the tools in this book and become more successful, your Grit Score will likely improve. Now, take this next line with a grain of salt because it is just our opinion (i.e., we don't have data to back this up), but if you notice your Grit Score declining over time, you may want to consider a more formal assessment for burnout. We are not prescribing this as a metric for everyone, but your mental health is important and you should use any tools available, even a silly Grit Score, to take stock of your psyche from time to time.

We have also briefly discussed Flow as being related to Deliberate Practice. But what is Flow? Mihaly Csikszentmihalyi answers that in his appropriately titled book, *Flow*. In this book, Dr. Csikszentmihalyi uses decades of his research to depict what flow is, why it's important, and how to reach it.

Using the Experience Sampling Method (ESM), Csikszentmihalyi asked his research participants to fill out a questionnaire at random times throughout the day. By compiling these data, he was able to identify how certain psychological constructs, such as boredom or anxiety, affect our state of being at any particular time. The ESM essentially provides a snapshot of what you are doing and how you feel about it in the moment.

Flow is a state where you are so engaged with a task that the rest of the world seems to disappear; where your mind, body, and soul are all temporarily in alignment. Although the concept is a little nebulous when written down, most people *do* have a sense of what we mean by this and experience flow states on a regular basis.

Csikszentmihalyi argues that, when at work, we usually reach Flow when our task is personally interesting and just difficult enough to challenge us to grow, without being so demanding that it induces worry/anxiety. The theory is that by consistently challenging yourself, you are striving for and reaching your goals. You are matching your task to your current skill set. Once you complete the task in front of you, it is time to progress to the next level of difficulty. And so on.

You may notice that this sounds *awfully similar* to the Growth Equation and to Deliberate Practice, which we discussed previously. This is not surprising. Many ideas from the self-help realm seem to overlap and point to the same eternal truths, just from slightly different perspectives, thus providing fresh reminders to busy adults.

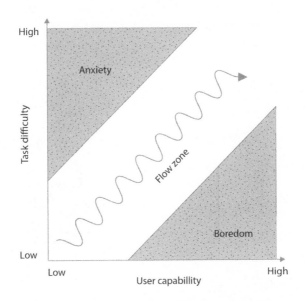

Being able to reach Flow in your studies will make the time fly and the study session seem much more manageable. If you are becoming overly stressed by your current study routine, you may be over-reaching. Pull back to a less anxiety-provoking schedule, if at all possible. Or vary your practice in new and more interesting ways.

If you can find autotelic ways to study – i.e., tasks that you find intrinsically interesting/motivating - then it is much easier to reach Flow. Keep developing, learning, building, and growing. If interested, you can also find free variations of the ESM questionnaire online, or find a phone app that will conduct the randomly timed notifications for you.

But before we try to rush into the Flow state, we should plan to get into the right preparatory mindset for our studies: cue *Eye of the Tiger!*

Understanding our existing mindset will also prove valuable when it comes to self-assessment and tailoring our habits for success. This notion has been made more popular by the book, *Mindset*, written by psychologist Carol Dweck. She focused on comparing the Growth Mindset to the Fixed Mindset. Her work primarily involved children, but her arguments should hold true for adult learners too.

Briefly, if a child has a **Fixed Mindset** they will assume that their more successful peers have "natural advantages" or were "born that way." In contrast, the **Growth Mindset** asserts that one shapes his/her own success by embracing the continuous process of self-improvement.

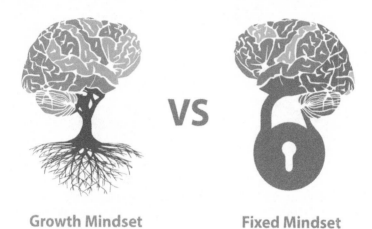

Growth Mindset	Fixed Mindset
I like learning new things.	I need to be good at something to enjoy it.
I push through my frustration.	Frustration makes me give up.
I like to be challenged.	I like staying in my comfort zone.
I learn from my mistakes.	When I fail, I feel like a failure.
I'm inspired by the success of others.	I'm threatened by the success of others.

Coping with failure and standing up to new challenges are par for the course in medical school. Fortunately, we know that it's within each person's power to shift his/her thinking from the Fixed Mindset to the Growth Mindset. For physicians, there's also research showing that encouraging their patients to embrace the Growth Mindset can improve health outcomes [78,79].

If interested, you can take your own Mindset Quiz [80]. See where you have room to improve. Then set your (SMART) goals, record your progress, and learn how to overcome any obstacle. Dweck would encourage you to focus on the process of growth, to enjoy your successes, but more importantly to embrace failures as learning opportunities; this is sometimes called *Failing Forward*.

Note from Chase: "After hitting several academic roadblocks, I was starting to think, 'maybe you're just not cut out for this.' However, by studying the theory of learning and trying out new study tactics, I was able to overcome many of my limiting beliefs."

Stress Mindset

Stress Mindset touches on or is related to, many themes in performance psychology, including the Growth Mindset, challenge mindset, approach motivation, loss aversion, and others. We all hate stress, right? It's bad for us, isn't it? Even the American Heart Association states that higher stress levels correlate with a higher risk of cardiovascular disease [81]. But without stress, we cannot grow.

While the amount of stress in our lives is important, our ability to cope with stressors is probably more important. This is where the Stress Mindset comes into play. Judging stressful stimuli as challenges to overcome instead of debilitating obstacles (i.e., having a positive Stress Mindset) seems to be correlated with lower burnout rates [82]. So, in reality, the best scenario is to be *eu-stressed* with a positive Stress Mindset.

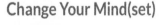

Change Your Mind(set)

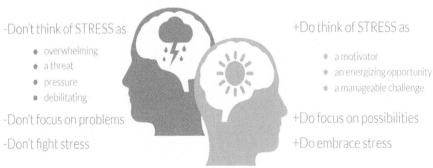

-Don't think of STRESS as
- overwhelming
- a threat
- pressure
- debilitating

-Don't focus on problems

-Don't fight stress

+Do think of STRESS as
- a motivator
- an energizing opportunity
- a manageable challenge

+Do focus on possibilities

+Do embrace stress

Resilience training is commonly used in sports psychology and medicine to help establish a positive Stress Mindset. A resilient person tends to face adversity with the old adage, "What doesn't kill me makes me stronger." Some who face traumatic events or stressful situations become overwhelmed and suffer. However, everyone has inherent strengths and weaknesses. Resilience training helps to produce better results by emphasizing the trainee's personal strengths and teaching skill sets that can help the trainee to overcome setbacks and life barriers [83,84].

How could we apply this to medical school? Well, in the same way that the Growth Equation (stress + rest = growth) requires physical stress for growth, our cognitive faculties need to be exercised to expand. In fact, stress under the right circumstances can enhance memory/retention [85]. To our knowledge, this model has not been directly studied in graduate-level students, but all three of us would assert that we grew tremendously during our graduate studies because of the stresses imposed upon us.

State & Self

EQ vs. IQ

At this point, the term **Emotional Intelligence** (EI or EQ) has become a part of the popular lexicon. In the mid-1990s, Dr. Daniel Goleman coined the term with his book, *Emotional Intelligence*, which produced a paradigm shift in the way psychologists viewed intelligence as a whole. Based on his research, Goleman hypothesized that EQ is actually more important than the traditional intelligence quotient (IQ) in leadership and other important areas of character development. Even with a remarkably high IQ, individuals with low EQ (on average) experience less success [86].

Though all medical students were over-achievers before starting MS1 - among the most gifted students in their undergraduate classes - they now find themselves in an environment where everyone else is just as (if not more) talented in the IQ department. Every medical student is also a hard worker. Realizing that *you're not so special* can be a shock to the ego. Dr. David Larson, the author of *Medical School 2.0*, expressed a similar sentiment when he was interviewed on the *Medical Mnemonist* podcast.

To stand out in medicine, you need to have a deep sense of emotional intelligence that allows you to establish therapeutic contact with your patients and goodwill among your colleagues. On average, women have higher EQ than men. Side note: female doctors were recently reported to have lower patient mortality rates than their male counterparts [87]. Hats off to the ladies!

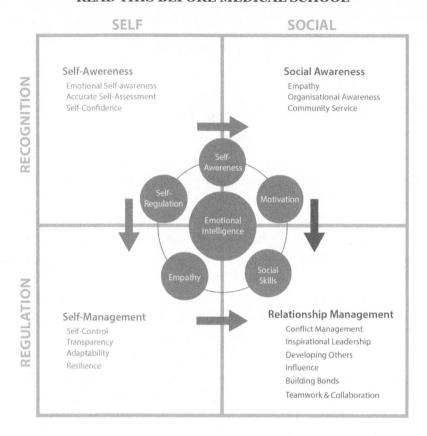

While some dispute Goleman's model of EQ [88], his ideas have been widely accepted by psychologists with some minor modifications [89-91]. In broad strokes, Goleman emphasized that there are 5 Categories of Emotional Intelligence. These consist of 1) self-awareness (for which Goleman advocates meditation), 2) self-regulation, 3) motivation, 4) empathy, and 5) social skills. Thankfully, all of these can be improved if you choose to put the work in.

When we start to pick up on our own internal thought patterns & emotions, we can then begin to redirect negative energy into productive action, similar to the psychological concept of *sublimation*. Further, when we have a keen eye for emotional distress in others, we can provide better support or guidance as needed.

So, whether it be in the classroom with students and instructors, or on the wards with patients and staff, developing EQ will be critical for any student doctor. Being resentful on rounds, condemning your peers, mistreating patients/staff, or venting on social media won't just harm your career, but it could harm patients. Begin to develop your EQ just like any other skill. You could even formulate a SMART goal, then Plan, Do, Study, Act.

There are many tests out there that claim to determine your EQ score, but to get a baseline assessment, we would recommend using validated instruments from the literature like the EQ-i 2.0 [92] or the Test for Emotional Intelligence (TIE) [90]. A free test can be found at PsychologyToday.com by typing "emotional intelligence test" into the search box, though they charge about ten dollars to see the detailed results [93].

So, what are some practical ways to improve your emotional intelligence? You could start by reading Goleman's book, *Emotional Intelligence*. One of the first steps he encourages is to begin a meditation practice, such as Mindfulness or Compassion meditation. We will discuss meditation a bit more in the section on Spiritual Health but if you want to jump right into it, we would recommend you check out the free courses offered by the Center for Mindfulness, based out of the University of Massachusetts School of Medicine [94].

Gratitude & Happiness

Mindfulness, gratitude, happiness are all cultural buzzwords these days. In the West, we seem to be deluded into thinking that, "if I just reach the next milestone or buy the next thing, then I can be grateful & happy." Even if we *intellectually* know this isn't the case, our behavior seems to suggest otherwise.

As a premed, you may have thought that earning a high GPA or crushing the MCAT would make you happy. Don't get us wrong, these are commendable achievements, but did the happiness last? For some, the answer may be yes, but we suspect that for most of the personalities drawn to medicine, these were simply more checkboxes to fill. Nothing really changes when you're in medical school, residency, and beyond. Crushing the USMLE or COMLEX does not provide any greater or longer-lasting sense of wellbeing than crushing the MCAT.

None of the authors of this book pretend to hold the *secrets* of happiness. At our very best, we are able to keep the important things in mind throughout the day, like our relationships with family, friends, colleagues, and patients. What is happiness? You may think you know, but philosophers, poets, and researchers have struggled to objectively define this human construct. How can we use data from the current scientific literature to benefit our studies, personal relationships, and professional lives?

For this topic, we could draw from a number of sources. Many of the books and articles on the psychology of happiness tend to revolve around a three-pronged construct consisting of pleasure, engagement, and meaning [95]. First, we intuitively know that, because pleasurable experiences are transient by nature, they are a necessary but insufficient mediator of happiness. Second, being an engaged member of our family, community, and workplace seems to be another core element of a happy life. Third, we spend a huge amount of our time working on our relationships and careers, so if we do not find meaning in these, then we are unlikely to find happiness. Taking a job primarily for the money or prestige is a recipe for burnout [96-98].

Throughout this book, we have emphasized the importance of self-assessment to track your progress. So, where could you go to get a baseline assessment of your psychological disposition? Consider filling out the free Via Survey at ViaCharacter.org [99]. This lengthy questionnaire is a positive psychology survey that, according to their website, assesses one's "love, teamwork, curiosity, gratitude, social intelligence, creativity, and self-regulation." If you're on a tight timeline, you could opt for the Satisfaction with Life Scale instead, which is a widely used 5-question instrument for studies related to positive psychology [100].

Even without taking questionnaires, you can immediately begin to implement happiness-boosting practices. The Positive Psychology Program [101] lists dozens of activities that can promote wellbeing. Some of these include keeping a Gratitude Journal, reframing situations to see obstacles as challenges (i.e., endorsing a positive Stress Mindset), minimizing negative verbiage in your speech, eliminating negative self-talk, exercising, eating right, meditating, and more.

In particular, Loving-Kindness Meditation (LKM) and Compassion Meditation have been shown to alleviate many kinds of psychological stressors [102]. In 2011, an interesting paper described that these compassion-based meditations were linked to decreased stress and enhanced activity in the areas of the brain related to emotional processing and empathy [102]. Further, a review of the literature suggested that LKM increases positive emotions overall [103], though more robust trials are needed to make firm conclusions. Directly relevant to (future) physicians: meditation can increase your sense of resilience and decrease your likelihood of burnout [104,105].

Happiness and gratitude often go hand-in-hand. So, what is gratitude? Robert Emmons and Robin Stern, authors of *Gratitude as a Psychotherapeutic Intervention* [106], believe that gratitude consists of 1) affirming that there are good things in one's life, and 2) recognizing that some sources of good are outside of oneself. Beyond psychological benefits for anxiety and depression, they found that practicing gratitude can lower blood pressure and even enhance immune responses.

Practicing gratitude cultivates well-being and happiness, as well as strengthening our resilience. While the benefits of gratitude take time to accumulate, the effects tend to persist. The topic has grown so much that UC Berkeley's Greater Good Science Center [107] has even created free online courses for the topic (which can be found through Class-central.com). To get the most out of your gratitude practice, you should plan to involve others. Begin with a close friend or family member. You can then slowly work your way up to more difficult relationships as your skills develop.

Confidence and Presence

We have a secret to share: we're frauds. Actually, let's rephrase that: we have all *felt* like frauds in the past, yet we have all been successful. All throughout undergrad, we had the lingering doubt: could I really get into med school? Then, can I really make it through the *rest* of medical school? Then, there's no way I could get through intern year, how could I possibly expect to finish residency?! And so on. This is **Imposter Syndrome**.

Imposter syndrome has been heavily reported on in recent years. It tends to affect more women than men, but men tend to experience more severe symptoms [108]. It is a notorious nemesis to the aspiring physician [109]. Imposter syndrome can strike at any time, like when sitting in your classroom, in preparation for an interview, or when taking care of a patient. Self-doubt produces tremendous anxiety, but it steadily regresses with time as you become an increasingly competent person and physician.

Dr. Amy Cuddy is a social psychologist who has explored the topic of confidence. In her research, she found a simple hack to help boost your confidence. It seems silly, but your body language not only describes your level of confidence, but it can actually reinforce your level of confidence [110,111]. Cuddy popularized this notion in her TED talk on "Power Poses". Expansive postures come naturally when individuals feel powerful, victorious, and confident. In contrast, a shrinking posture signals self-doubt, weakness, and impotence.

Not only are there psychological effects of Power Posing, but Cuddy's lab found physiologic effects of too. A simple 1-minute power stance increased testosterone and lowered cortisol levels [112], which exert a wide range of biological effects. Dr. Cuddy explores this idea further in her book, *Presence*. If you're intrigued, consider reading her book, watching the TED talk, or simply testing out your power stance before the next exam, speech, or interview. What's the harm?

Physical Health

When dealing with such complex topics as physical health and nutrition, we could write a series of books and still only scratch the surface. And even if we knew everything there was to know about these topics, there is no one-size-fits-all solution. However, the **common-sense basics will apply to everyone**. You need to exercise, get enough sleep, and eat a well-balanced diet that consists of a variety of fresh foods. Minimize your intake of processed foods and moderate your consumption of alcohol and caffeine. Thus far, all of this is obvious to a future doctor, but we think there are some helpful points to elaborate on in this section.

First, it's important to know, especially when it comes to nutrition, that its science and medicine have a shaky past. The term "evidence-based medicine" was only recently coined in the 1990s and, although the concept of the double-blind randomized controlled trial dates back to (at least) the 1830s [113], proper RCTs of nutrition have not been widely implemented. When studying diet and nutrition, it is remarkably challenging to perform rigorous studies that provide high-quality evidence to support any definitive conclusions. Mostly because of funding limitations, nutrition studies have been riddled with problems like small sample sizes, self-report data, poor dietary adherence, short intervention duration, losses to follow-up, etc. As a result, studies are often mixed or even contradictory.

On top of all that, food can be a politically-charged topic and various industries muddy the water with lobbying efforts and less-than-rigorous research methodologies. Without going too far down that endless pit of historical confusion, let's break this section up into a few main points: physical activity, modern nutritional science, and sleep. Understanding that there is no "perfect state" for any of these categories will also benefit you. Shoot for incremental positive changes, or Kaizen.

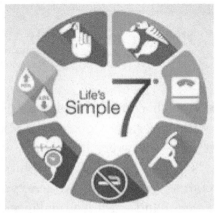

Source: American Heart Association.

To help easily disseminate information to the masses, a few organizations have provided simple dietary rules and checklists to guide patients and physicians. The American Heart Association developed *Life's Simple 7* to provide their recommendations on the most beneficial activities one can take for heart health. These seven steps include increasing activity level, eating a balanced diet, controlling cholesterol levels, controlling blood pressure, losing weight, reducing blood sugar, and quitting smoking.

The American Institute for Cancer Research (AICR), in partnership with the World Cancer Research Fund, has also made recommendations in recent years. Their Interactive Matrix [114] allows visitors to visualize the types of foods that may lead to protective or harmful cancer outcomes. Their *Continuous Update Report* is a global research project on nutrition and physical activity as these relate to cancer [115]. For the most part, AICR recommendations are in agreement with the American Heart Association.

It seems that everyone wants to generically prescribe more exercise and better diets. In fact, this is something physicians are notorious for doing without providing specific recommendations. This can lead to confusion, non-compliance, and distrust of the traditional medical establishment.

The best way to advise our future patients about these basic healthy lifestyle habits is to walk-the-walk, so we can thoughtfully describe how to go about exercising, eating, and sleeping well. Not only will it be of vital importance for comprehensive patient care, but proper exercise and nutrition can decrease mental illness [116,117], improve memory [118], prevent neurodegenerative disease [119], attenuate inflammatory disease [120], and even speed recovery in stroke victims [121].

In the world of exercise/fitness, there is always something new and trendy, but we all know that it really comes down to moving your body more. The first hurdle is to get started; then you need to keep going. Use any tools or lines that you can, in order to get your patients (and yourself) to buy-in to regular exercise. Then you can start to think about designing a fitness program. Any fitness program can be structured using the acronym, FITT (frequency, intensity, time, type). See a few examples in the table below.

FITT	Interval Training	Resistance Training	Endurance Training	Passive Physical Therapy
Frequency	3-7 times/week	3-5 times/week	3-7 times/week	3-7 times/week
Intensity	Moderate (40-59% VO2peak, up to 85%); Short (30 sec)	Low (lightweight); 10 reps/small muscle groups	Moderate (40-59% VO2peak)	Passive
Time	10-30 min	Up to 30 min	60 min	30 min
Type	Bicycle	Dumbbells	Walking	Stretching, breathing, relaxation

Ideally, we could all get at least 75 minutes of vigorous aerobic activity per week, or 150 minutes of moderate-intensity exercise, or a combination of the two. But if you *genuinely* don't have the time, then you could consider alternative strategies like one found in Tim Ferriss' popular book, *The 4 Hour Body*. Ferriss advocates for shorter periods of high-intensity interval training (HIIT) training, even just a few minutes per day. Check out his Talk at Google for a summary of his arguments [123].

HIIT has gained substantial popularity in the general public. It has also caught the eye of sports scientists and rehabilitation medicine, so we have studies supporting its use. For example, HIIT has been shown to reduce subcutaneous fat nine-times better than regular endurance training [124] and it doubled cardiorespiratory fitness compared to moderate aerobic exercise [125]. HIIT has also been shown to improve cardiovascular health and decrease markers of metabolic disease [125].

However, not everyone can go from couch potato to HIIT athlete in a single day. In fact, it may be dangerous to transition too quickly. We all have that friend who tried jumping straight into CrossFit and hurt themselves [126]. Regardless of your starting point, if you want your fitness level to climb, it's important to continue pushing yourself just beyond your comfort level when exercising. Then, after being worn out by a good exercise bout, allow your body to rest with a good night's sleep. Remember the growth equation: stress + rest = growth.

While exercise is great, you cannot neglect nutrition. Thankfully, there are many validated tools we can use to evaluate and guide our food choices. The Healthy Eating Index is an assessment of what most Americans eat and how it compares to key recommendations set forth by the US Department of Agriculture [127,128].

The recommendations used for the HEI reflect conventional wisdom: increase the amount and variety of fresh fruits and vegetables, whole grains, and high-quality protein, while also decreasing sugar, fat, and salt content. Though this may seem like common sense to healthcare workers, it could be just the right thing for your stubborn hypertensive patient who loads up his microwave dinner steak and potatoes with salt, and then washes it all down with a cold beer (or six)!

Additionally, the Diet Quality Index International (DQI-I) is a validated measure of how diet quality varies between countries [129]. It focuses on five factors in human diets: the variety of food groups, the variety of protein sources, adequate intake of high-quality foods (fruits & veggies), moderation of non-essential foods, and the balance of macronutrients. Less than 40% of the U.S. population achieves adequate vegetable intake and only 16% have an adequate intake of fiber [130]. Further, Americans scored poorly in sodium content and fats consumed (ratios of unsaturated to saturated fats). Taken altogether, America scores 59% out of 100% on the DQI-I.

As a nation, we fail at nutrition. But many *individual* Americans are trying to make positive changes to their lives. Your future patients will have many questions for you, including questions about fad diets. So, we thought it would be worthwhile to provide some commentary about contemporary diets.

Low-Carb: Low-carbohydrate diets increase the daily intake of fat and protein to make up for the loss of carbohydrates. Carbs are the easiest macronutrient to absorb. Low-carb diets do show greater weight loss and better cholesterol control in the short-term [131], however one-year follow-up showed no significant differences in weight loss [132,133], which is a pretty consistent pattern seen for long-term weight loss diets in general.

Ketogenic: Ketogenic diets are the most extreme kind of low carb diet. Theoretically, by cutting out all carbs (and lowering overall caloric intake), you can suppress insulin production and this allows our cells to burn more fatty acids for energy. At the same time, the liver starts to produce ketones in an attempt to spare the limited amount of glucose in the blood for the tissues that really need it: the brain and red blood cells. In effect, by cutting out all carbs, you are trying to trick your body into thinking that it is fasting (at least from the perspective of the major hormones that control cell metabolism, like insulin, glucagon, cortisol, and thyroid hormone).

Though users of the ketogenic diet will often swear by it, to our knowledge there have been no high-quality, long-term studies that demonstrate its ability to keep the weight off or to improve overall health. Like most other diets, any weight changes are usually short-term while the subject sticks closely to the diet, but the effects fade as they become less rigid with their food intake.

So, we cannot fully endorse the ketogenic diet for the general population, but in healthcare we are able to use ketogenic diets for a very specific purpose: drug-resistant forms of childhood epilepsy. We still don't know exactly why this works to prevent seizures, but there's pretty substantial evidence supporting its use [134,135].

Paleo: The main problem with the "paleolithic diet" is that experts don't seem to agree on exactly what foods would reflect the dietary patterns of antiquity [136]. In theory, it's supposed to consist of foods that one would find in pre-farming civilization, so it avoids items like grains, legumes, dairy, processed foods, added salt, and refined sugar. But it's hard to know exactly how we could make this work for the average person in today's industrialized world. Though some studies show favorable effects on metabolic health and blood pressure [137], the quality of the evidence is generally poor.

Mediterranean: The Mediterranean diet puts an emphasis on high consumption of fresh fruits and vegetables, whole grains, and healthy fats from olive oil, nuts, and fish. It is a popular alternative diet that appears to extend lifespan [138], prevent cardiovascular disease [139], slow age-related cognitive decline [140], and produce a healthier gut microbiome [141]. That's a whole lot of bang for your buck!

DASH: The Dietary Approach to Stop Hypertension (DASH) diet is very similar to the Mediterranean diet, focusing on increased fruits and vegetables, while also decreasing saturated fats and salt intake. In addition to lowering blood pressure [142], the DASH diet has been associated with decreased mortality [143], decreased bone thinning [144], as well as decreased heart disease and stroke in certain populations [145].

Weight Watchers: When it comes to weight loss, Weight Watchers is probably one of the most well-known names. It focuses on portion control and food tracking, more than simply avoidance of certain food groups. Programs like Weight Watchers also provide lots of social support which can make the decisive difference for long-term weight loss [146,147].

Mindful Eating: Bringing mindfulness to the dinner table is a relatively new but growing practice in the US. Mindful Eating is the simple act of paying much closer attention to the entire experience of eating: smell, taste, texture, sound, internal sensations, etc. It gets you to slow down and appreciate the subtleties inherent to the eating experience. But when you're engaging in mindfulness, remember that it is a process-driven behavior rather than a goal-oriented behavior [148]. That being said, some research into this area has linked mindful eating to better weight control [149].

To close out this section, we should mention that making lifestyle changes is hard for any person to do alone. Support groups and allied health professionals like Registered Dietitians or Personal Trainers can be a huge help in this area. We could all benefit from learning to take advantage of the ample resources around us.

Beyond Basic Nutrition and Exercise

Dr. Michael Greger is a controversial figure in the health and wellness scene [150]. For years, he has advocated for *everyone* to consume a whole-food, plant-based diet. Even if the health benefits of his diet are not as wide-reaching as he claims, increasing your consumption of fruits, vegetables, and whole-grains - while also decreasing consumption of animal products and processed foods - is *unlikely* to hurt the vast majority of people.

Greger's videos and podcasts on NutritionFacts.org cover a host of health-related problems, and his even more popular book, *How Not to Die*, delves into the science behind a diet centered on plant-based, whole-foods. If we were to condense the decades of research Dr. Greger draws from, it might look something like this:

Though there are still many unanswered questions regarding nutrition and dietary patterns, a plant-based whole-food diet might be the best choice for individuals aiming to control their weight, limit their risk of cardiovascular disease and diabetes, as well as decrease their chances of colorectal cancer [151-154]. Whole foods, which are unprocessed and as close to their natural form as possible, tend to be the healthiest choices in the supermarket.

Food processing strips food of nutrient-dense components like husks, shells, skins, etc. For example, exclusive consumption of polished rice is classically associated with thiamine deficiency, resulting in Beri Beri [155]. When fruits and vegetables are flash-frozen or prepared in other ways that destroy plant-specific enzymes, we may lose the nutrients that would have been created by those enzymes [156]. Plant-based foods, in general, have the highest density of nutrients per calorie when compared to animal products. Hence, the recommendation for plant-based whole foods. To simplify his recommendations, Dr. Greger has created the Daily Dozen, which you can see at his website [157].

High consumption of green leafy vegetables and fruits are at the top of many health-conscious individuals' minds. But what about nuts, beans, and spices? Each of these are packed with flavor and healthy micronutrients [158]. Beans are a great source of plant-based protein and fiber. Nuts are high in healthy fats and have been shown to improve satiety with meals and thereby limit weight gain [159].

If this seems like just another doctor-sponsored fad diet, it is important to note that many of the recommendations made in Dr. Greger's materials overlap nicely with those made in the Continuous Update Project of the American Institute for Cancer Research, which is a well-respected authority on the relationships between nutrition, everyday health, and cancer risk. For example, high red meat consumption is a well-known risk factor for colon cancer and cardiovascular disease. But if the same nutrients, like high-quality protein, can be obtained by plant-based means (e.g., beans & rice), why not consider replacing the potential carcinogen? Unfortunately, we are undereducated about the details of diet, nutrition, exercise, etc.

during our medical training, which makes it harder for us to make recommendations with confidence.

For rock-solid information on diet and nutrition, many Registered Dietitians turn to Krause's Food & The Nutrition Care Process. This would also be a great resource for interested physicians. While it certainly espouses a more conservative view than Dr. Greger, this reference book has great things to say about plant-based whole food diets. No matter what resources you choose, we recommend that you start thinking about how you can use your knowledge of lifestyle interventions early in your career. Many patients will have questions about the day-to-day features of a healthy lifestyle (especially nutrition & exercise), so you ought to have some practical tips to share!

Up to this point, we talked enough about exercise and nutrition, but what about **sleep**? We spend about one third of our lives in this state, so we ought to know something about it! Starting with the basics, most **adults need 7-9 hours** of quality sleep each night for optimal health [160]. But many medical students feel that they cannot spend this much time away from studying, so they forego sleep for their studies.

There's plenty of research to show that foregoing sleep to cram for your tests is a poor choice because sleep is essential for memory acquisition and consolidation [161, 162]. Sleep deprivation has been well studied. It is associated with poor academic performance [163], decreased work performance and attention span [164], and enormous economic costs (estimated to be in the tens of billions of dollars among western nations) [165]. Not only that, but sleep deprivation is hazardous to your health! A study of over 5 million individuals showed that less than 6 hours of sleep was associated with increased mortality in those with underlying health problems [166].

For those suffering from insufficient sleep, there are a number of non-pharmacologic tools that can be used. Exercise, relaxation practice, stimulus control, and good sleep hygiene (i.e., regular sleeping patterns, avoiding bright screens at bedtime, and abstaining from coffee and alcohol in the evening) can dramatically improve your sleep quality [167]. If these common-sense tactics don't work, consider seeking expert advice from your primary care provider who may then refer you to a sleep specialist.

If you're in the DIY mood, you could also try tracking your sleep with apps and wearables like the FitBit. The Department of Veteran Affairs offers a free cognitive behavioral therapy app for insomnia that could help to guide you towards better sleep hygiene [168].

Spiritual Health

Spiritual health is another amorphous topic that we ought to address. Some find it in church or prayer, some in hiking or gardening, and others by volunteering. However, the focus of this section will be on meditation because there is a growing interest among researchers and the general public. There's a wide range of options to choose from for the aspiring meditator, such as mindfulness, mantras, visualization, breathing, countdowns, relaxing scenes or background sounds, and more.

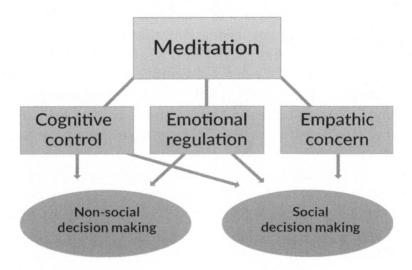

Although many people have tried to formally describe the exact experiences and benefits of meditation for the mind, their descriptions can come across as vague or mysterious. We've found that meditation is the kind of thing that each person needs to experience for themselves, rather than trying to rely on second-hand descriptions.

From a scientific standpoint, one of the best descriptions of the evidence base supporting the use of meditation can be found in *Altered Traits* by Daniel Goleman (also the author of *Emotional Intelligence*) and Richard Davidson (professor and close colleague of the Dalai Lama). Goleman and Davidson consolidated decades of research and personal experiences into their book.

Prior to publication, Goleman and Davidson found that much of the meditation research was poorly crafted. In fact, only about 1% of the thousands of meditation studies they reviewed matched the "gold standards" for scientific research, so they opted to use a more standardized program of Mindfulness-Based Stress Reduction (MBSR) for the sake of objectivity and consistency [169]. Their rigorous research, combined with work from many others in the field, provides strong support for the use of meditation for everyday wellbeing. Meditation may even stave off age-related cognitive decline [170].

The most common styles of meditation in the Western world are Mindfulness meditation (MM) and Transcendental meditation (TM). MM includes the subcategories of breathing techniques, body scans, insight, and loving-kindness meditation, while TM mainly consists of performing silent mantras. MM and TM are probably the easiest techniques for newbies to explore, requiring as little as 1-2 sessions per day lasting a few minutes each. That being said, both *Altered Traits* and a 2014 systematic review by the Journal of the American Medical Association suggest that MM has a stronger evidence base than TM [171].

There are interesting historical controversies and philosophical quibbles that arose between the advocates of different camps of meditation, but the bottom line is that you can find many different ways to incorporate this healthy practice into your life. For more information, we would direct you to the Insight Meditation Center website.

Regardless of the type of meditation you practice, it's important to anticipate the changes to your mental state that you may experience. The two types are State (temporary) and Trait (permanent) changes. Most people want to emphasize the Trait changes, but understanding the State changes is equally important.

It is vital to your practice to pay attention to the many small/temporary changes to your state of consciousness during mindfulness meditation. As you accumulate experience with sensing "internal" State changes, you'll also start to notice some of the "external" Trait changes. Research by Goleman and Davidson emphasizes this point: the more you practice, the more you benefit.

They also emphasize that, like diet and exercise, meditation is not a quick-fix. Meditation requires time and discipline to accumulate the reward.

When thinking about the changes that take place with meditation, we can also categorize them as Structural changes vs. Functional changes in the brain. Past research had assumed that any potential benefit from meditation was purely functional, like stress reduction or increased compassion and empathy. These functional changes are mediated by neurochemical/hormonal responses in the brain, and even the immune system plays a role [172].

Based on our current models of the brain, structure and function are inextricably linked, so any functional changes of the mind will coincide with structural changes in the brain. According to Dr. Goleman, these changes likely take place in structures like the nucleus accumbens and amygdala. But we have already gone down this rabbit hole far enough. If you're interested in starting meditation right away, you could check out an app like Headspace or you could try some of our basic recommendations on mindfulness (below).

Find a quiet and comfortable place. Many regular meditators have a specific room, chair, and time for their meditation practice. Sticking to the same routine and location can make it easier to continue your practice over time. Be willing to experiment with style. What works for someone else might not work for you.

To begin your practice, get comfortable. You can do the cross-legged Burmese style or just find a comfortable chair and have your feet flat on the ground. You can leave your eyes open at first and take in a few slow, deep breaths. With each exhalation, let your muscles relax and your mind calm. Start with a 5-minute session, then increase by 1-5 minute increments every few days with a goal of 20 minutes per day. The key is consistency of practice.

Now, the confusing part. Many people will assume that the goal is to have "a clear mind" and not to allow thoughts to intrude themselves into your stream of consciousness during meditation. Not true. There is no way to *stop* the thoughts. Mindfulness meditation is best explained in the passive sense:

"let it go" instead of "force it away." Trying to force anything in meditation is like trying to hold back the tide. Accept the thoughts that arise, then let them go and drift back to the center.

If these Mindfulness basics aren't working for you, don't get discouraged. Try to find another style or maybe a mentor who can guide your practice. Like getting a second medical opinion, you can always get multiple opinions on meditation. You could even try meditating under different circumstances like walking (Awe Walks [173]) or eating (Mindful Eating [174]).

Before we finish this section, one note about meditation wearables. Wearables are popular for exercise because they give immediate feedback in the moment. Though not the *end-all-be-all* for meditation practices, some wearables have demonstrated surprising usefulness.

For example, the Muse EEG headband has been featured in several scholarly articles. It has been used to verify that mindfulness practice improved the attention span of study participants [175]. It has also been used as an affordable alternative to other portable EEG machines in detecting event-related brain potentials [175]. This device works by sending a signal to your phone to play a sound when the EEG detects an electrical pattern consistent with a "wandering" mind. Another cool feature is that the phone app is gamified to give participants more points for more time in "calmer" meditative states.

No matter your starting point, if you want a practice that is likely to decrease your stress, anxiety, depression, and burnout as well as lead to a host of other physical and psychological benefits, meditation is a great way to go. It can improve your study attention and mood [176], improve your patient interaction [177,178], and reduce testing anxiety [179]. Like anything else, it all depends on how much you put into it.

Leadership and Branching Out

"Management is doing things right;
leadership is doing the right things."
Peter F. Drucker

Leadership is often entirely overlooked in our medical curriculum. It is assumed that all medical students have mastered leadership traits and skills, but few of us receive formal training. Fully dissecting the theory and styles of leadership would take an entire course, but it is important for physicians to know and internalize the basics. Learning how to act, interact with peers and staff, and find solutions to problems are universally useful skills. Even as a student, you have probably seen the value of a good leader when completing group projects, where getting everyone moving in the same direction can feel like herding cats.

A contemporary model of leadership that we have found valuable is Transformational Leadership. A transformational leader actively works with employees and team members to foster greater productivity by leveraging the inherent talents and creativity of their team members (rather than micromanaging and exploiting). Transformational leaders tend to be self-motivated, direct, intelligent, confident, and honest. The New England Journal of Medicine also added good communicator, empathic, and emotionally intelligent to the list [180].

If you need additional motivation, strong leadership skills will be important from the perspective of your future residency program directors and your future healthcare administrators. About one-sixth of your future workload will be consumed by administrative work (rather than direct patient care) [181], so it will be critical to not only develop your clinical skills but also your business skills. Focusing on your leadership can have a "spillover effect" that is directly relevant to being an effective businessperson [182].

If you wish to test your leadership abilities and style, there are a number of assessments that have been developed. These include the Transformational Leadership Survey, the Leadership Practices Inventory, and the Collaborative Leadership Self-Assessment Questionnaire, among others. Unfortunately, you have to pay for many of these. For training, a great place to start may be your school's Career Services office. The American College of Physicians offers free webinars and purchasable leadership courses on their ACP Leadership Academy page [183]. There are also a host of resources on the Education page of the Physician Leaders website [184] and Medscape Physician Business Academy [185].

For those who wish to stay in healthcare but find clinical medicine to not be the best fit, there are also many great sites that provide inspiration and guidance. The Physician Non-Clinical Careers website [186] and the Drop-Out Club [187] offer ideas and training for a variety of non-clinical science and medicine-based occupations. For those looking to go into nonprofit entrepreneurial work, another resource is the Society of Physician Entrepreneurs [188]. They offer biomedical and healthcare innovation opportunities for physicians looking to branch into new areas.

As a busy medical student (or pre-med), it is perfectly acceptable to focus your energies on the present to crush your classes. However, being aware that these resources and options exist can do wonders for your stress levels. Many students feel locked into a particular path and fearful of what would happen if that single path were taken away. Know that there are communities out there, training available, and countless options available to you. You are smart. You are hardworking. You will succeed.

Ethics

Medical ethics is a mandatory part of the curriculum in medical school, so the material presented in this section will only survey items that are not covered in a typical medical ethics class, such as **Leadership Ethics** and **Effective Altruism**. Broad strokes will suffice to give the subject attention and to prompt interested learners towards further reading.

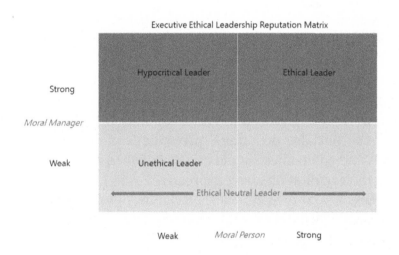

In managerial and business circles, the Ethical Leadership Matrix is an easy-to-visualize depiction of what makes a proper leader (see image above). In the seminal paper, *Moral Person and Moral Manager* [189], Trevino et al. present their findings from dozens of interviews with managers and business leaders on the topic of Ethical Leadership. They argue that one must gain a *reputation* for being ethical; it is not enough to simply behave ethically in your private life. The Moral Manager gains a favorable reputation by Modeling good behavior, by fairly dispensing Rewards and Discipline, and by Communicating their ethics/values.

Consistently showing weakness as a Moral Person and Moral

Manager produces the reputation of an Unethical Leader. Being a strong Moral Manager and weak Moral Person classifies one as a Hypocritical Leader. Being a strong Moral Person and weak Moral Manager is left Undefined. And, of course, being strong in both earns one the coveted title of an Ethical Leader. Great... but why does this matter to medical students and physicians?

Most have heard about the Enron and Worldcom scandals, which spurred moral outrage on behalf of the wider business community. However, it is not just big Wall Street firms that behave unethically. There are plenty of examples of improper financial behavior in healthcare, implicating organizations such as the Veterans Affairs Administration [190-192], mental health institutions [193,194], and individual hospitals [195,196].

These ethical lapses degrade public trust in the medical establishment. Had the leaders of these organizations strived for Ethical Leadership, by behaving transparently and ensuring appropriate checks/balances were in place, they could have avoided all the negative publicity (and its downstream consequences on patient care). Ethical leadership is based, not just on your own character traits, but also on others' perceptions of you, so medical professionals and companies should reinforce habits and policies that help to keep their reputation above reproach.

Being aware of your own ethical shortcomings - we all have them - is a step towards self-improvement. One way to assess your personal ethics is through the Ethical Lens Inventory [197]. The creator of the inventory, Professor Cathyrn Byrd, J.D., developed it based on 10+ years of research and testing.

The inventory has been used by over 600,000 individuals in a wide variety of businesses. It has even been used by hospital systems for leadership ethics training. The Ethical Lens Inventory can help you determine where you lie on certain ethical boundaries and it provides input on how you can broaden your ethical understanding.

Interestingly, in a private correspondence, Dr. Byrd suggested that one of the reasons clashes often occur between physicians and nurses regarding patient care is due to their Ethical Lenses. In general, physicians take a more consequentialist stance, while nurses tend to have a more deontological perspective. She posits that because these moral positions differ so much, physicians and nurses are often in disagreement about what actions are in the best interest of the patient. Many healthcare systems will try to strike a balance between consequentialist and deontological ethics by focusing on how to provide cost-effective approaches that also provide the highest quality of care to each individual patient.

If you're interested in these sorts of ethical discussions, then you probably wonder how your career will help to make a positive impact on the world. In their Guide to a Fulfilling Job [198], the 80,000 Hours group has put together a very unique way to assess how we can actually "do the most good" with our career. If interested in the topic, you could visit their website or check out the *Doing Good Better Podcast*, hosted Dr. William MacAskill.

It is perfectly acceptable to discover that the "traditional" pathway of earning the MD or DO immediately followed by a career in clinical medicine is not right for you. You don't need to join Doctors Without Borders in order to do good. Every effort that's taken in good faith will count for something, but with some careful analysis, you can find ways to maximize your impact on humanity.

Perhaps research or academics is a better fit than clinical medicine. You may find that an administrative position is the best place to help out the entire hospital system. Or maybe you decide to make as much money as possible in order to maximally donate to thoughtful charities. One organization that does a great job of vetting charities is called GiveWell.org. Check out their website for more information.

Closing Thoughts - Part 1

As we mentioned in the Home Study section, it is important to immediately start using the tactics and techniques discussed thus far. Just get started, anywhere you're able. If you cannot apply them right away, make sure to take notes on the important features relevant to you (and plan to revisit those notes later). Obviously, don't let our tips on personal development get in the way of your studies. Use what you can and be adaptable. Good things are sure to follow.

There are massive physical, emotional, and psychological benefits to dedicated self-improvement, but it's also important to recognize when you need some outside help. If you're unsure of where to go, or if things get out of hand and you don't feel safe, please reach out to one of these free services.

1) National Alliance on Mental Illness Helpline: 1-800-950-NAMI (6264)

2) National Suicide Prevention Lifeline: 1-800-273-TALK (8255)

3) 24/7/365 Crisis Hotline: Call 1 (800) 273-8255

4) Crisis Text Link: Text "HOME" to 741741

5) Depression/Anxiety Hotline: 866-229-5544

6) Substance Abuse and Mental Health Services Administration Helpline: 1-800-662-HELP (4357)

7) Better Help Online Counseling Service: contact@betterhelp.com

References - Part 1

References can also be found at https://freemeded.org/book-references/

1. Croston G. (2012) The thing we fear more than death: why predators are responsible for our fear of public speaking. URL: https://www.psychologytoday.com/us/blog/the-real-story-risk/201211/the-thing-we-fear-more-death
2. Esposito J. Conquering stage fright. URL: https://adaa.org/understanding-anxiety/social-anxiety-disorder/treatment/conquering-stage-fright
3. Densen P. (2011) Challenges and opportunities facing medical education. URL: https://www.ncbi.nlm.nih.gov/pmc/articles/PMC3116346/
4. Dyrbye LN et al. (2008) Burnout and suicidal ideation among US medical students. URL: https://annals.org/aim/article-abstract/742530/burnout-suicidal-ideation-among-u-s-medical-students
5. Morris NP. (2016) If healthcare providers can't overcome the stigma of mental illness, who will? URL: https://www.washingtonpost.com/opinions/if-health-care-providers-cant-overcome-the-stigma-of-mental-illness-who-will/2016/05/20/993eca46-1dfd-11e6-9c81-4be1c14fb8c8_story.html?noredirect=
6. (2017) Understanding Learning and Attention Issues. URL: https://www.ncld.org/news/state-of-learning-disabilities/understanding-learning-and-attention-issues#ch1howcommon
7. (2015) Mental Disorders and Disabilities Among Low-Income Children: 16. Prevalence of Learning Disabilities. URL: https://www.ncbi.nlm.nih.gov/books/NBK332880/
8. Baserra V et al. (2017) On-task and off-task behavior in the classroom: A study on mathematics learning with educational video games. URL: https://journals.sagepub.com/doi/abs/10.1177/0735633117744346
9. Godwin KE et al. (2016) Off-task behavior in elementary school children. URL: https://www.sciencedirect.com/science/article/pii/S0959475216300275
10. Bradbury NA. (2016) Attention span during lectures: 8 seconds, 10 minutes, or more? URL: https://www.physiology.org/doi/full/10.1152/advan.00109.2016
11. Hope V & Henderson M. (2014) Medical student depression, anxiety and distress outside North America: a systematic review. URL: https://www.ncbi.nlm.nih.gov/pubmed/25200017
12. Azad N et al. (2017) Anxiety and depression in medical students of a private medical college. URL: https://www.ncbi.nlm.nih.gov/pubmed/28712190
13. (2015) Ergonomics. URL: https://www.ehs.harvard.edu/programs/ergonomics
14. Bhattacharya A. (2014) Costs of occupational musculoskeletal disorders (MSDs) in the United States. URL: https://www.cdc.gov/niosh/nioshtic-2/20044181.html
15. Ergonomics: Tools & Guides. URL: https://www.navfac.navy.mil/products_and_services/sf/products_and_services/ergonomics/tools_guides.html
16. Shrestha N et al. (2016) Workplace interventions for reducing sitting at work. URL: https://www.cochrane.org/news/health-effects-sit-stand-desks-and-interventions-aimed-reduce-sitting-work-are-still-unproven
17. Finch LE et al. (2017) Taking a stand: The effects of standing desks on task performance and engagement. URL: https://www.ncbi.nlm.nih.gov/pmc/articles/PMC5580641/
18. Computer vision syndrome. URL: https://www.aoa.org/patients-and-public/caring-for-your-vision/protecting-your-vision/computer-vision-syndrome
19. Novotney A. (2011) Silence, please: Psychologists are increasing awareness of the harmful effects noise has on cognition and health. URL: https://www.apa.org/monitor/2011/07-08/silence.aspx
20. Vardy M. Why noise is better than quiet. URL: https://www.lifehack.org/articles/productivity/why-noise-is-better-than-quiet.html
21. Verified signatories of the IFCN code of principles. (Updated 2020) URL:

https://ifcncodeofprinciples.poynter.org/signatories

22. Goodman J et al. (2019) Heat and learning. URL: https://www.nber.org/papers/w24639

23. Oswald CJP et al. (2010) Disruption of comprehension by the meaning of irrelevant sound. URL: https://www.tandfonline.com/doi/abs/10.1080/09658210050117762

24. Rosen LD. (2013) Phantom pocket vibration syndrome. URL: https://www.psychologytoday.com/us/blog/rewired-the-psychology-technology/201305/phantom-pocket-vibration-syndrome

25. Dixon T. (2019). 10 Cardinal rules for surviving first year. URL: https://www.amsa.org/2017/08/09/10-cardinal-rules-surviving-first-year/

26. Lopez RB et al. (2018) Media multitasking is associated with altered processing of incidental, irrelevant cues during person perception. URL: https://www.ncbi.nlm.nih.gov/pmc/articles/PMC6180433/

27. Lee M et al. (2015) Interaction with indoor plants may reduce psychological and physiological stress by suppressing autonomic nervous system activity in young adults: A randomized crossover study. URL: https://www.ncbi.nlm.nih.gov/pmc/articles/PMC4419447/

28. Nieuwenhuis et al. (2014) The relative benefits of green versus lean office space: Three field experiments. URL: https://psycnet.apa.org/record/2014-30837-001

29. Atchley RA & Strayer DL. (2012) Creativity in the wild: Improving creative reasoning through immersion in natural settings. URL: https://journals.plos.org/plosone/article?id=10.1371/journal.pone.0051474

30. Sisti HM et al. (2007) Neurogenesis and the spacing effect: Learning over time enhances memory and survival of new neurons. URL: https://www.ncbi.nlm.nih.gov/pmc/articles/PMC1876761/

31. Spalding KL et al. (2013) Dynamics of hippocampal neurogenesis in adult humans. URL: https://www.cell.com/cell/fulltext/S0092-8674(13)00533-3?_returnURL=https%3A%2F%2Flinkinghub.elsevier.com%2Fretrieve%2Fpii%2FS0092867413005333%3Fshowall%3Dtrue

32. Tashiro A et al. (2007) Experience-specific functional modification of the dentate gyrus through adult neurogenesis: A critical period during an immature stage. URL: https://www.jneurosci.org/content/27/12/3252

33. Pan SC. (2015) The interleaving effect: Mixing it up boosts learning. URL: https://www.scientificamerican.com/article/the-interleaving-effect-mixing-it-up-boosts-learning/

34. Carvalho PF & Goldstone RL. (2014) Effects of interleaved and blocked study on delayed test of category learning generalization. URL: https://www.ncbi.nlm.nih.gov/pmc/articles/PMC4141442/

35. Karpicke JD. (2016) A powerful way to improve learning and memory: Practicing retrieval enhances long-term, meaningful learning. URL: https://www.apa.org/science/about/psa/2016/06/learning-memory.aspx

36. Kelly P & Whatson T (2013) Making long-term memories in minutes: a spaced learning pattern from memory research in education. URL: https://www.ncbi.nlm.nih.gov/pmc/articles/PMC3782739/

37. Oakley B & Sejnowski T. (Updated 2020) Learning how to learn: Powerful mental tools to help you master tough subjects. URL: https://www.coursera.org/learn/learning-how-to-learn

38. The Learning Scientists website. (Updated 2020) URL: http://www.learningscientists.org/

39. Abdulmouti H. (2018) The benefits of Kaizen to business excellence: Evidence from a case study. URL: https://www.omicsonline.org/open-access/benefits-of-kaizen-to-business-excellence-evidence-from-a-case-study-2169-0316-1000251-104386.html

40. Dhand S. (2014) Pareto's principle in hospital medicine. URL: https://www.medscape.com/viewarticle/835473

41. Schmidt et al. (2016) Classroom-based physical activity breaks and children's attention: Cognitive engagement works! URL: https://www.ncbi.nlm.nih.gov/pmc/articles/PMC5047899

42. Popeska et al. (2018) Implementation of Brain Breaks in the classroom and effects on attitudes toward physical activity in a Macedonian school setting. URL: https://www.ncbi.nlm.nih.gov/pmc/articles/PMC6025620/

43. (Updated 2020) Meditation: A simple, fast way to reduce stress. URL:

https://www.mayoclinic.org/tests-procedures/meditation/in-depth/meditation/art-20045858

44. (Updated 2015) Health literacy universal precautions toolkit, 2nd edition: Plan-Do-Study-Act (PDSA) directions and examples. URL: https://www.ahrq.gov/professionals/quality-patient-safety/quality-resources/tools/literacy-toolkit/healthlittoolkit2-tool2b.html

45. Dyrbye L & Shanafelt T (2016) A narrative review on burnout experienced by medical students and residents. URL: https://www.ncbi.nlm.nih.gov/pubmed/26695473

46. Hätinen M et al. (2007) Comparing two burnout interventions: Perceived job control mediates decreases in burnout. URL: https://www.researchgate.net/publication/211387089_Comparing_Two_Burnout_Interventions_Perceived_Job_Control_Mediates_Decreases_in_Burnout

47. Steinberg BA et al. (2016) Feasibility of a mindfulness-based intervention for surgical intensive care unit personnel. URL: https://www.ncbi.nlm.nih.gov/pubmed/27965223

48. Ayala EE et al. (2017) Prevalence, perceptions, and consequences of substance use in medical students. URL: https://www.ncbi.nlm.nih.gov/pmc/articles/PMC5678442/

49. Goodman M & Berlinerblau M (2018) Discussion: Treating burnout by addressing its causes. URL: https://www.physicianleaders.org/news/discussion-treating-burnout-by-addressing-its-causes

50. Panesar et al. (2009) The WHO checklist: A global tool to prevent errors in surgery. URL: https://www.ncbi.nlm.nih.gov/pmc/articles/PMC2693116/

51. Haynes et al. (2009) A surgical safety checklist to reduce morbidity and mortality in a global population. URL: https://www.nejm.org/doi/full/10.1056/NEJMsa0810119

52. Carroll RG (2017) In the valley of the blind, the USMLE is king. URL: https://www.physiology.org/doi/full/10.1152/advan.00021.2017

53. Mehta NB et al. (2016) More on how USMLE Step 1 scores are challenging academic medicine. URL: https://journals.lww.com/academicmedicine/Fulltext/2016/05000/More_on_How_USMLE_Step_1_Scores_Are_Challenging.3.aspx

54. Prober CG et al. (2016) A plea to reassess the role of USMLE Step 1 scores in residency selection. URL: https://www.ncbi.nlm.nih.gov/pubmed/26244259

55. Armstrong A et al. (2007) Do USMLE Step 1 scores correlate with council on resident education in OBGYN in-training examination scores and American Board of Obstetrics and Gynecology written examination performance? URL: https://www.ncbi.nlm.nih.gov/pubmed/17615848

56. Murphy B (Updated 2020) USMLE Step 1 moves to pass-fail: Answers to 7 key questions. URL: https://www.ama-assn.org/residents-students/usmle/usmle-step-1-moves-pass-fail-answers-7-key-questions

57. Deci EL et al. (1999) A meta-analytic review of experiments examining the effects of extrinsic rewards on intrinsic motivation. URL: http://psycnet.apa.org/record/1999-01567-001

58. Karson M (2014) The myth of intrinsic motivation: It's undignified to get caught working for superficial rewards. URL: https://www.psychologytoday.com/us/blog/feeling-our-way/201401/the-myth-intrinsic-motivation

59. Froiland JM et al. (2012) Intrinsic motivation to learn: The nexus between psychological health and academic success. URL: https://link.springer.com/article/10.1007/BF03340978

60. Newton PM (2015) The learning styles myth is thriving in higher education. URL: https://www.ncbi.nlm.nih.gov/pmc/articles/PMC4678182/

61. Forrin ND & MacLeod CM (2017) This time it's personal: The memory benefit of hearing oneself. URL: https://www.tandfonline.com/doi/abs/10.1080/09658211.2017.1383434?journalCode=pmem20)https://www.ncbi.nlm.nih.gov/pmc/articles/PMC3268356/

62. Abrous DN & Wojtowicz JM (2015) Interaction between neurogenesis and hippocampal memory system: New vistas. URL: https://cshperspectives.cshlp.org/content/7/6/a018952.full

63. Jiang L et al. (2016) Cortical thickness changes correlate with cognition changes after cognitive training: Evidence from a Chinese community study. URL: https://www.ncbi.nlm.nih.gov/pmc/articles/PMC4877512/

64. Leonard M et al. (2004) The human factor: The critical importance of effective teamwork and communication in providing safe care. URL:

https://www.ncbi.nlm.nih.gov/pmc/articles/PMC1765783/

65. (Updated 2020) Misinformation effect. URL: https://en.wikipedia.org/wiki/Misinformation_effect

66. Ozbay F et al. (2007) Social support and resilience to stress: From neurobiology to clinical practice. URL: https://www.ncbi.nlm.nih.gov/pmc/articles/PMC2921311/

67. Molero Jurado MDM et al. (2018) Burnout risk and protection factors in certified nursing aides. URL: https://www.ncbi.nlm.nih.gov/pubmed/29848982

68. Merino-Plaza MJ et al. (2018) Burnout in the staff of a chronic care hospital. URL: https://www.ncbi.nlm.nih.gov/pubmed/29723388

69. Duan X et al. (2019) The impact of workplace violence on job satisfaction, job burnout, and turnover intention: The mediating role of social support. URL: https://www.ncbi.nlm.nih.gov/pubmed/31146735

70. Carron AV et al. (1985) The development of an instrument to assess cohesion in sport teams: The Group Environment Questionnaire. URL: https://journals.humankinetics.com/doi/pdf/10.1123/jsp.7.3.244

71. Whitton SM & Fletcher RB (2013) The Group Environment Questionnaire: A multilevel confirmatory factor analysis. URL: https://journals.sagepub.com/doi/abs/10.1177/1046496413511121?journalCode=sgrd&

72. Collaborative Intelligence (CQ) Checklist. URL: http://content.randomhouse.com/assets/9780812994919/view.php?id=collint001

73. Zwarenstein M et al. (2009) Interprofessional collaboration: Effects of practice based interventions on professional practice and healthcare outcomes. URL: https://www.cochranelibrary.com/cdsr/doi/10.1002/14651858.CD000072.pub2/abstract

74. Roughead RE et al. (2009) The effectiveness of collaborative medicine reviews in delaying time to next hospitalization for patients with heart failure in the practice setting. URL: https://www.ahajournals.org/doi/full/10.1161/CIRCHEARTFAILURE.109.861013

75. Dr. Amy Wrzesniewski Faculty Page, Yale School of Management (Updated 2020). URL: https://som.yale.edu/faculty/amy-wrzesniewski

76. Brooks K (2012) Job crafting: Turning the job you have into the job you want. URL: https://www.psychologytoday.com/us/blog/career-transitions/201207/job-crafting

77. Dr. Angela Duckworth's Grit Scale. URL: https://angeladuckworth.com/grit-scale/

78. Crum A (2017) Changing mindsets to enhance treatment effectiveness. URL: https://mbl.stanford.edu/sites/g/files/sbiybj9941/f/crum_zuckerman_jama_2017.pdf

79. (2017) Analysis: Making mindset matter. URL: https://www.bmj.com/content/356/bmj.j674

80. Mindset Quiz. URL: http://homepages.math.uic.edu/~bshipley/MindsetQuiz.w.scores.pdf

81. American Heart Association. (2014) Stress and heart health. URL: https://www.heart.org/en/healthy-living/healthy-lifestyle/stress-management/stress-and-heart-health

82. Ben-Avi N et al. (2018) "If stress is good for me, it's probably good for you too": Stress mindset and judgment of others' strain. URL: https://www.researchgate.net/publication/319873843_If_stress_is_good_for_me_it's_probably_good_for_you_too_Stress_mindset_and_judgment_of_others'_strain

83. Fletcher D & Sarkar M. (2016) Mental fortitude training: An evidence-based approach to developing psychological resilience for sustained success. URL: https://www.tandfonline.com/doi/full/10.1080/21520704.2016.1255496?scroll=top&needAccess=true

84. Forbes S & Fikretoglu D. (2018) Building resilience: The conceptual basis and research evidence for resilience training programs. URL: https://journals.sagepub.com/doi/pdf/10.1037/gpr0000152

85. Cahill L et al. (2003) Enhanced human memory consolidation with post-learning stress: Interaction with the degree of arousal at encoding. URL: https://www.ncbi.nlm.nih.gov/pmc/articles/PMC202317/

86. Goleman, D. (2006). *Emotional Intelligence*.

87. Tsugawa Y et al. (2017) Comparison of hospital mortality and readmission rates for Medicare

patients treated by male vs. female physicians. URL: https://jamanetwork.com/journals/jamainternalmedicine/fullarticle/2593255

88. Cherniss C et al. (2010) Emotional intelligence: What does the research really indicate? URL: https://www.tandfonline.com/doi/abs/10.1207/s15326985ep4104_4

89. Romanelli F et al. (2006) Emotional intelligence as a predictor of academic and/or professional success. URL: https://www.ncbi.nlm.nih.gov/pmc/articles/PMC1636947/

90. Smieja M et al. (2014) TIE: An ability Test of Emotional Intelligence. URL: https://journals.plos.org/plosone/article?id=10.1371/journal.pone.0103484

91. Drigas AS & Papoutsi C. (2018) A new layered model on Emotional Intelligence. URL: https://www.ncbi.nlm.nih.gov/pmc/articles/PMC5981239/

92. EQ-i-2.0 URL: http://www.eiconsortium.org/measures/eqi.html

93. PsychologyToday Emotional Intelligence Test. URL: https://www.psychologytoday.com/us/tests/personality/emotional-intelligence-test

94. UMass Center for Mindfulness. URL: https://www.umassmed.edu/cfm/

95. Vella-Brodrick DA et al. (2009) Three ways to be happy: Pleasure, Engagement, and Meaning - Findings from Australian and US samples. URL: https://www.jstor.org/stable/27734781?seq=1

96. Pasricha N. (2016) Avoid burnout by asking this question. URL: https://hbr.org/2016/06/avoid-burnout-by-asking-this-question

97. Mayo Clinic Staff (2018) Job burnout: How to spot it and take action. URL: https://www.mayoclinic.org/healthy-lifestyle/adult-health/in-depth/burnout/art-20046642

98. Deci EL et al. (1991) Motivation and education: The self-determination perspective. URL: http://selfdeterminationtheory.org/SDT/documents/1991_DeciVallerandPelletierRyan_EP.pdf

99. Via Character Survey. URL: http://viacharacter.org/

100. Satisfaction with Life Scale. URL: http://www.midss.org/content/satisfaction-life-scale-swl

101. Ackerman CE. (Updated 2020) What is positive mindset: 89 ways to achieve a positive mental attitude. https://positivepsychologyprogram.com/positive-mindset/#activities-positive-mindset

102. Hofmann SG et al. (2011) Loving-Kindness and Compassion Meditation: potential for psychological interventions. URL: https://www.ncbi.nlm.nih.gov/pmc/articles/PMC3176989/

103. Fredrickson BL et al. (2008) Open hearts build lives: Positive emotions induced through Loving-Kindness meditation, build consequential personal resources. URL: https://www.ncbi.nlm.nih.gov/pmc/articles/PMC3156028/#R48

104. Seppala EM et al. (2014) Loving-Kindness Meditation: a tool to improve healthcare provider compassion, resilience, and patient care. URL: https://jcompassionatehc.biomedcentral.com/articles/10.1186/s40639-014-0005-9

105. Beollinghaus I et al. (2012) The role of mindfulness and loving-kindness meditation in cultivating self-compassion and other-focused concern in healthcare professionals. URL: https://self-compassion.org/wp-content/uploads/publications/LKMnursesupdate.pdf

106. Emmons RA & Stern R. (2013) Gratitude as a psychotherapeutic intervention. URL: http://ei.yale.edu/wp-content/uploads/2013/11/jclp22020.pdf

107. UC Berkeley Greater Good Science Center. URL: https://greatergood.berkeley.edu/

108. Badawy RL et al. (2018) Are all imposters created equal? Exploring gender differences in the impostor phenomenon-performance link. URL: https://www.sciencedirect.com/science/article/abs/pii/S0191886918302435

109. Russell R. (2017) On overcoming imposter syndrome. URL: https://journals.lww.com/academicmedicine/fulltext/2017/08000/On_Overcoming_Imposter_Syndrome.12.aspx

110. Carney DR et al. (2010) Power posing: Brief nonverbal displays affect neuroendocrine levels and risk tolerance. URL: http://web.missouri.edu/~segerti/capstone/powerposing.pdf

111. Cuddy AJ et al. (2015) Preparatory power posing affects nonverbal presence and job interview performance. URL: https://psycnet.apa.org/doiLanding?doi=10.1037%2Fa0038543

112. Cuddy AJ et al. (2012) The benefits of power posing before a high-stakes social evaluation. URL: https://dash.harvard.edu/bitstream/handle/1/9547823/13-027.pdf?sequence=1

113. Stolberg M (2016) Inventing the randomized double-blind trial: The Nurnberg salt test of 1835. URL: https://www.jameslindlibrary.org/articles/inventing-the-randomized-double-blind-trial-

the-nurnberg-salt-test-of-1835/

114. World Cancer Research Fund, Interactive Cancer Risk Matrix (Updated 2020) URL: https://www.wcrf.org/dietandcancer/interactive-cancer-risk-matrix

115. American Institute for Cancer Research, Continuous Update Project (Updated 2020) URL: https://www.aicr.org/continuous-update-project/

116. Mikkelsen K et al. (2017) Exercise and mental health. URL: https://www.sciencedirect.com/science/article/abs/pii/S0378512217308563

117. Marx W et al. (2017) Nutritional psychiatry: the present state of the evidence. URL: https://www.ncbi.nlm.nih.gov/pubmed/28942748

118. Godman H. (Updated 2018) Regular exercise changes the brain to improve memory, thinking skills. URL: https://www.health.harvard.edu/blog/regular-exercise-changes-brain-improve-memory-thinking-skills-201404097110

119. Duzel E et al. (2016) Can physical exercise in old age improve memory and hippocampal function? URL: https://academic.oup.com/brain/article/139/3/662/2468800

120. Beavers KM et al. (2010) Effect of exercise training on chronic inflammation. URL: https://www.ncbi.nlm.nih.gov/pmc/articles/PMC3629815/

121. Saunders DH et al. (2014) Physical activity and exercise after stroke. URL: https://www.ahajournals.org/doi/10.1161/STROKEAHA.114.004311

122. Mayo Clinic Healthy Lifestyle (Updated 2019) URL: https://www.mayoclinic.org/healthy-lifestyle/fitness/expert-answers/exercise/faq-20057916

123. Tim Ferriss Talk at Google on HIIT. URL: https://www.youtube.com/watch?v=hpv4h_B2n6k

124. Tremblay A et al. (1994) Impact of exercise intensity on body fatness and skeletal muscle metabolism. URL: https://www.sciencedirect.com/science/article/pii/0026049594902593

125. Weston KS et al. (2013) High-intensity interval training in patients with lifestyle induced cardiometabolic disease: A systematic review and meta-analysis. URL: https://bjsm.bmj.com/content/48/16/1227.short

126. Smith MM et al. (2013) Crossfit-based high intensity power training improves maximal aerobic fitness and body composition. URL: https://g-se.com/uploads/blog_adjuntos/crossfit_based_high_intensity_power_training_improves_maximal_aerobic_fitness_and_body_composition..pdf

127. USDA Healthy Eating Index. URL: https://www.cnpp.usda.gov/healthyeatingindex

128. Wilson MM et al. (2016) American diet quality: Where is it, where is it heading, and what could it be? URL: https://www.ncbi.nlm.nih.gov/pmc/articles/PMC4733413/

129. Newby PK et al. (2003) Reproducibility and validity of the Diet Quality Index Revised as assessed by use of a food frequency questionnaire. URL: https://academic.oup.com/ajcn/article/78/5/941/4677503

130. Soowon K et al. (2003) The Diet Quality Index International provides an effective tool for cross-national comparison of diet quality as illustrated by China and the United States. URL: https://academic.oup.com/jn/article/133/11/3476/4817926

131. Yancy WS et al. (2004) A low carbohydrate, ketogenic diet vs. a low fat diet to treat obesity and hyperlipidemia: A randomized controlled trial. URL: https://annals.org/aim/fullarticle/717451

132. Foster GD et al. (2003) A randomized trial of low carbohydrate diet for obesity. URL: https://www.nejm.org/doi/full/10.1056/nejmoa022207

133. Gardner CD et al. (2018) Effect of low fat vs. low carbohydrate diet on 12-month weight loss in overweight adults and the association with genotype pattern or insulin secretion. URL: https://jamanetwork.com/journals/jama/fullarticle/2673150

134. Epilepsy Society Page on Ketogenic Diet. URL: https://www.epilepsysociety.org.uk/ketogenic-diet

135. Martin-McGill KJ et al. (2018) Ketogenic diets for drug-resistant epilepsy. URL: https://www.cochranelibrary.com/cdsr/doi/10.1002/14651858.CD001903.pub4/full

136. Mayo Clinic Healthy Lifestyle (Updated 2017) URL: https://www.mayoclinic.org/healthy-lifestyle/nutrition-and-healthy-eating/in-depth/paleo-diet/art-20111182

137. Frassetto LA et al. (2009) Metabolic and physiologic improvements from consuming a paleolithic, hunter-gatherer type diet. URL: https://www.nature.com/articles/ejcn20094

138. Estruch R et al. (2013) Primary prevention of cardiovascular disease with a Mediterranean diet. URL: https://www.nejm.org/doi/full/10.1056/nejmoa1200303

139. Romagnolo DF & Selmin OI. (2017) Mediterranean diet and prevention of chronic diseases. URL: https://www.ncbi.nlm.nih.gov/pmc/articles/PMC5625964/

140. Valls-Pedret C et al. (2015) Mediterranean diet and age-related cognitive decline. URL: https://jamanetwork.com/journals/jamainternalmedicine/fullarticle/2293082?gtmRefSection=Enfermedades-y-Condiciones

141. De Filippis F et al. (2015) High-level adherence to a Mediterranean diet beneficially impacts the gut microbiota and assocated metabolome. URL: https://gut.bmj.com/content/65/11/1812.short

142. Sacks FM et al. (2001) Effects on blood pressure of reduced dietary sodium and the Dietary Approaches to Stop Hypertension diet. URL: https://www.nejm.org/doi/full/10.1056/nejm200101043440101

143. Parikh A et al. (2009) Association between a DASH-like diet and mortality in adults with hypertension: Findings from a population-based follow up study. URL: https://academic.oup.com/ajh/article/22/4/409/155233

144. Lin P et al. (2003) The DASH diet and sodium reduction improve markers of bone turnover and calcium metabolism in adults. URL: https://academic.oup.com/jn/article/133/10/3130/4687581

145. Fung TT et al. (2008) Adherence to a DASH-style diet and risk of coronary heart disease and stroke in women. URL: https://jamanetwork.com/journals/jamainternalmedicine/article-abstract/414155

146. Truby H et al. (2006) Randomised controlled trial of four commercial weight loss programmes in the UK: initial findings from the BBC "diet trials". URL: https://www.bmj.com/content/332/7553/1309?grp=1

147. American Psychological Association: How social support can help you lose weight. URL: https://www.apa.org/topics/obesity/support

148. Nelson JB. (2017) Mindful eating: The art of presence while you eat. URL: https://www.ncbi.nlm.nih.gov/pmc/articles/PMC5556586/

149. Lofgren IE. (2015) Mindful eating: An emerging approach for healthy weight management. URL: https://journals.sagepub.com/doi/abs/10.1177/1559827615569684

150. Hall H. (2013) Death as a foodborne illness curable by veganism. URL: https://sciencebasedmedicine.org/death-as-a-foodborne-illness-curable-by-veganism/

151. Oxford Vegetarian Study. URL: http://www.epic-oxford.org/oxford-vegetarian-study/

152. Wright N et al. (2017) The BROAD study: A randomised controlled trial using a whole food plant-based diet in the community for obesity, ischemic heart disease or diabetes. URL: https://www.nature.com/articles/nutd20173

153. Crowe FL et al. (2011) Diet and risk of diverticular disease in Oxford cohort of European prospective into cancer and nutrition. URL: https://www.ncbi.nlm.nih.gov/pmc/articles/PMC3139912/

154. Le LT & Sabate J. (2014) Beyond meatless, the health effects of vegan diets: Findings from the Adventist cohorts. URL: https://www.ncbi.nlm.nih.gov/pmc/articles/PMC4073139/

155. Wikipedia: Thiamine deficiency. URL: https://en.wikipedia.org/wiki/Thiamine_deficiency

156. Vermeulen M et al. (2008) Bioavailability and kinetics of sulforaphane in humans after consumption of cooked versus raw broccoli. URL: https://www.ncbi.nlm.nih.gov/pubmed/18950181

157. Dr. Greger's Daily Dozen. URL: https://nutritionfacts.org/daily-dozen-challenge/

158. Pagan CN. (Updated 2019) Spices and herbs that can help you stay healthy. URL: https://www.webmd.com/healthy-aging/over-50-nutrition-17/spices-and-herbs-health-benefits

159. Tan SY et al. (2014) A review of the effects of nuts on appetite, food intake, metabolism, and body weight. URL: https://academic.oup.com/ajcn/article/100/suppl_1/412S/4576547

160. Watson WF et al. (2015) Recommended amount of sleep for a healthy adult: A joint consensus statement of the American Academy of Sleep Medicine and Sleep Research Society. URL: https://jcsm.aasm.org/doi/10.5664/jcsm.4758

161. National Institute of Neurological Disorders and Stroke. (Updated 2019) Brain Basics:

Understanding Sleep. URL: https://www.ninds.nih.gov/Disorders/Patient-Caregiver-Education/Understanding-Sleep

162. Division of Sleep Medicine at Harvard Medical School. (Updated 2007) Sleep, learning, and memory. URL: http://healthysleep.med.harvard.edu/healthy/matters/benefits-of-sleep/learning-memory

163. Phillips AJK et al. (2017) Irregular sleep/wake patterns are associated with poorer academic performance and delayed circadian and sleep/wake timing. URL: https://www.nature.com/articles/s41598-017-03171-4

164. National Sleep Foundation. A good night's sleep helps with job performance. URL: https://www.sleepfoundation.org/excessive-sleepiness/performance/good-nights-sleep-helps-job-performance

165. Hillman D et al. (2018) The economic cost of inadequate sleep. URL: https://www.ncbi.nlm.nih.gov/pubmed/29868785

166. Itani O et al. (2016) Short sleep duration and health outcomes: A systematic review, meta-analysis, and meta-regression. URL: https://www.sciencedirect.com/science/article/pii/S1389945716301381?via%3Dihub

167. National Sleep Foundation. What is sleep hygiene? URL: https://www.sleepfoundation.org/articles/sleep-hygiene

168. VA Cognitive Behavioral Therapy Coach app. URL: https://www.mobile.va.gov/app/cbt-i-coach

169. Goleman D & Davidson R.J. (2018) Altered Traits: Science Reveals How Meditation Changes Your Mind, Brain, and Body

170. Khalsa DS & Perry G. (2017) The four pillars of Alzheimer's prevention. URL: https://www.ncbi.nlm.nih.gov/pmc/articles/PMC5501038/

171. Goyal M et al. (2014) Meditation programs for psychological stress and well-being: A systematic review and meta-analysis. URL: https://jamanetwork.com/journals/jamainternalmedicine/fullarticle/1809754?alert=article

172. Jindal V et al. (2013) Molecular mechanisms of meditation. URL: https://www.ncbi.nlm.nih.gov/pubmed/23737355

173. Greater Good Science Center. Awe Walk. URL: https://ggia.berkeley.edu/practice/awe_walk

174. Nelson JB (2017) Mindful eating: The art of presence while you eat. URL: https://www.ncbi.nlm.nih.gov/pmc/articles/PMC5556586/

175. Krigolson OE et al. (2017) Choosing MUSE: Validation of a low-cost portable EEG system for ERP research. URL: https://www.ncbi.nlm.nih.gov/pmc/articles/PMC5344886/

176. Bhayee S et al. (2016) Attentional and affective consequences of technology supported mindfulness training: A randomised, active control, efficacy trial. URL: https://www.ncbi.nlm.nih.gov/pmc/articles/PMC5127005/

177. Beach MC et al. (2013) A multicenter study of physician mindfulness and healthcare quality. URL: https://www.ncbi.nlm.nih.gov/pmc/articles/PMC3767710/

178. Amutio-Kareaga A et al. (2017) Improving communication between physicians and their patients through mindfulness and compassion-based strategies: A narrative review. URL: https://www.ncbi.nlm.nih.gov/pmc/articles/PMC5373002/

179. Cho H et al. (2016) The effectiveness of daily mindful breathing practices on test anxiety of students. URL: https://journals.plos.org/plosone/article?id=10.1371/journal.pone.0164822

180. Rihal CS. (2017) The importance of leadership to organizational success. URL: https://catalyst.nejm.org/importance-leadership-skills-organizational-success/

181. Woolhandler S & Himmelstein DU. (2014) Administrative work consumes one-sixth of US physicians' working hours and lowers their career satisfaction. URL: https://www.ncbi.nlm.nih.gov/pubmed/25626223

182. Sogunro OA. (1997) Impact of training on leadership development: Lessons from a leadership training program. URL: https://journals.sagepub.com/doi/abs/10.1177/0193841X9702100605

183. American College of Physicians Leadership Academy. URL: https://www.acponline.org/meetings-courses/acp-courses-recordings/acp-leadership-academy

184. Physician Leaders Education Page. URL: https://www.physicianleaders.org/education

185. Medscape Physician Business Academy. URL: https://www.medscape.com/academy/business

186. Physician Non-Clinical Careers website. URL: https://www.nonclinicalcareers.com/

187. Drop Out Club website. URL: https://www.docjobs.com/

188. Society of Physician Entrepreneurs website. URL: https://www.sopenet.org/

189. Trevino LK et al. (2000) Moral person and moral manager: How executives develop a reputation for ethical leadership. URL: http://homepages.se.edu/cvonbergen/files/2012/12/Moral-Person-and-Moral-Manager_How-Executives-Develop-a-Reputation-for-Ethiccal-Leadership1.pdf

190. VA hospital scandal article 1. URL: https://www.washingtonpost.com/politics/2018/11/13/four-years-after-scandal-va-gets-praise-health-care-falls-short-access/?noredirect=on

191. VA hospital scandal article 2. URL: https://www.vox.com/2014/9/26/18080592/va-scandal-explained

192. VA hospital scandal article 3. URL: https://www.usatoday.com/story/news/usanow/2014/06/23/phoenix-va-whistleblower/11297069/

193. Mental health facility scandal 1. URL: https://www.nytimes.com/1991/11/24/us/paying-for-fraud-special-report-mental-hospital-chains-accused-much-cheating.html

194. Mental health facility scandal 2. URL: https://www.beckershospitalreview.com/legal-regulatory-issues/9-connecticut-psych-hospital-employees-charged-in-patient-abuse-scandal.html

195. Individual hospital scandal 1. URL: https://www.latimes.com/archives/la-xpm-2008-aug-05-me-health5-story.html

196. Individual hospital scandal 2. URL: https://www.washingtonpost.com/local/md-politics/maryland-hospital-system-under-fire-for-self-dealing/2019/03/15/b8140f12-472b-11e9-8aab-95b8d80a1e4f_story.html?noredirect=on&utm_term=.8423559a7a20

197. Ethical lens inventory page. URL: https://studylib.net/doc/8765553/understanding-the-ethical-lens-inventory

198. 80,000 Hours Group website. URL: https://80000hours.org/book/

PART 2: TEST PREPARATION AND EXAM DAY

"Winners never quit, and quitters never win."
Vince Lombardi

Pre-Test: On a scale of 1-7 (1 = never and 7 = always) rate these questions.

#	Question/Statement	SCORE
1	Prior to each exam, I have an established preparation plan.	/7
2	I always know the number of questions, time limitations, and other exam rules for the assessment I am about to take.	/7
3	I understand the "anatomy" of a board-style question and can use this to determine what the question writer would like me to know.	/7
4	I focus on the quality of my test-taking practice more than the quantity.	/7
5	I use the MedEdge Method for tackling test questions.	/7
	TOTAL	/35

Finally, the section many of you have been waiting for. Perhaps this is your sole reason for purchasing our book. Here we answer the question, "What are the main concerns when it comes to test-taking in medical school?" Of course, we have covered study tips to help prepare you for this content. We have covered the healthy mind and body to make sure we are in peak (or at least fair) physical and mental condition. Further, you are aware of the lessons gleaned by much of the modern literature on educational psychology and neuroscience.

Now it is time to dissect test questions and discuss the current best-practices for overcoming obstacles on test day. The literature on student examinations - particularly for medical students taking the boards - does not paint a very clear picture of how exactly to prepare. Generally, the more practice questions you complete, the higher your score [1]. But beyond that simple correlation, there isn't much consensus on specific steps you can take to improve your scores. So, with this chapter, we will draw upon our experience to provide you with a solid strategy to prepare for your board exams.

Students studying for the bar exam or their CPA accreditation are told that their exams are difficult. And we're sure they are. But medical boards are a different animal. The USMLE Step 1 and COMLEX Level 1 require the student to actively deconstruct hundreds of questions for hours on end, and to synthesize the information from thousands of in-class hours to come up with the right answer. Not to mention the information is inherently complex and constantly being updated. It takes intelligence, diligence, and endurance to perform well.

The USMLE Step exams (MD) and the COMLEX Level exams (DO) are designed to assess your overall medical knowledge in the fairest way possible. Medicine is becoming increasingly complicated, so doctors these days need to work hard to keep up with the latest advancements in their field. In a similar manner, medical students need to use an up-to-date test-taking strategy when approaching the boards.

Your fellow students and even instructors may chant the ever-popular mantra, "Do more questions!" While this is partially correct, learning from board-style practice questions can be made much more effective when you have an insider's perspective on how the questions are designed.

In this section, we will focus on how to decipher the question vignette and **get into the mindset of a test writer**. By taking this perspective, you will see how the vignette tries to direct you in a particular direction to produce the right answer. We will also cover a method that helps you to keep track of the key details, to avoid distracters, and to whittle down the answer choices. Practicing and believing in your premade strategy - whether you get the answer right or wrong - will greatly reduce your stress levels going into the test. In our experience, less stress means more confidence and better exam performance. Let's get started!

Dissecting a Boards Question

Rather than trying to intuitively pick up the patterns behind board questions with massed study, why not learn about them ahead of time? Let's start with the basics. A boards-style question is comprised of a question **vignette** (question stem), a **question** (an interrogatory or "lead-in question"), and **answer choices**.

The vignette may be as short as a few sentences or may contain several paragraphs-worth of information, including patient history, presentation, physical exam findings, lab results, imaging, and any other pertinent information. The interrogatory asks a question that, despite occasionally seeming ambiguous, is designed to have a **single best answer**. So far, so good?

There will generally be 5 answer choices, but you may see questions with up to 12. Several will be obviously incorrect, while others are designed to trap students with common mistakes. The test-writer's manual flat out states that there should be 3 to 5 distractors among the answer choices. Sneaky little devils, aren't they?

Most questions will have a relatively straightforward correct answer (if you know the material well enough). This is referred to as the **cover the options rule**, whereby a student should be able to cover the answer choices and still come to the correct answer without first looking at the options. It should not be ambiguous. But in reality, many questions will come down to a hard choice between 2-3 options.

Test writers - both on the boards and at your school - also like to recycle well-written question stems to assess your complete knowledge of a topic. This can be something as simple as changing the interrogatory from "what is the diagnosis if X happens" to "what is the diagnosis if Y happens." Alternatively, they may change it from a single-step diagnosis question to a question that requires two logical inferences to answer, referred to as a **two-step question**.

An example of a two-step question could look something like this: the vignette states that a guy has "a tall, thin body habitus with elongated fingers" and is complaining of "vision problems." You may quickly associate these findings with an underlying diagnosis of

Marfan Syndrome. But the interrogatory asks something like, "Which of the following best describes the inheritance pattern of his underlying disease?" (For the record, Marfan's is inherited in an autosomal dominant pattern.) So, you would need to take two-steps to get this question correct: 1) his constellation of signs and symptoms suggests Marfan Syndrome, and 2) Marfan's is inherited in an autosomal dominant fashion.

On the boards, it is rarely as straightforward as: Question > Diagnosis. More often you will see two-step questions like: Question > Diagnosis > Treatment (or biochemical pathway, expected lab test results, associated findings on imaging or histology, etc.). Sometimes they will hit you with a three-step question to *really* plumb the depths of your understanding.

History of the NBME, NBOME, USMLE, and COMLEX Exams

To properly prepare for the boards, it will help to know a little bit about the organizations responsible for writing them. At the very least, we can better understand the test from the perspective of the test writers. Like Sun Tzu said, it's best to *know your enemy...* or your examiner.

The National Board of Medical Examiners (NBME) was created in 1915 to produce one nationally recognized medical licesnsing exam. This is known as the United States Medical Licensing Exam (USMLE). Prior to this, every state administered different board exams with different requirements. As you can imagine, this inconsistency between states was problematic. Nowadays, it is required for all allopathic (MD) medical students to pass the full series of USMLE exams (Steps 1, 2, 3, and the Clinical Skills exam) to practice medicine in the United States. The USMLE is also voluntarily taken by many osteopathic (DO) students, but osteopaths have their own analogous set of exams to take.

If you want reliable information about the boards, just go straight to the USMLE website produced by the NBME, rather than relying on hearsay from your classmates. They even freely provide the NBME Item Writing Guide (The Gold Book) to help direct your faculty on how to write fair test questions. You can also find useful information about how to prepare, including subject matter breakdowns, free practice questions, and full-length practice exams.

The National Board of Osteopathic Medical Examiners (NBOME) is the osteopathic student's equivalent to the NBME. Founded in 1934, the NBOME aims to be a "Global Leader in the Assessment of Osteopathic Medicine & Related Health Care Professions." The NBOME writes the DO equivalent to the USMLE, known as the Comprehensive Osteopathic Medical Licensing Exam (COMLEX).

In the past, osteopathic students would take their COMLEX and apply to a residency designed specifically for DOs. Most allopathic residency programs recognized the COMLEX as a truly equivalent test to the USMLE, but not all programs held this view. So, if a DO student wanted to go to an allopathic residency (or if they simply wanted to keep their options open), then that student would elect to take the USMLE Step 1, in addition to the COMLEX. Thankfully, the two residency tracks (MD and DO) are being merged into a single graduate medical education system, which should help to simplify things in the world of GME.

How to Approach and Prepare for the Boards

How should you think about the boards? How should you prepare? These are important questions that every student asks. The answer is pretty simple, but the execution is difficult. You already have everything it takes to prepare for and dominate the USMLE or COMLEX.

It's important to note here that you can read every USMLE blog and forum out there (e.g., Student Doctor Network), which will fill you with anxiety about the exam and leave you confused about how to proceed with your studies. Try not to stress out about what these blogs and forums say because there is little-to-no data, that is both vetted and publicly available, on how best to prepare for the test. Most of the information you'll see is based on self-reported experience. We recommend that you find a resource you trust, put together a game plan that you can stick to, and then play your own game. DO NOT compare yourself to others!

Also, try your hardest - though this may feel impossible - to not worry about your exam scores. The board exams were intended to be a demonstration of basic medical competency, and should still be viewed that way. Although many students think their Step score is the *only* important part of their application, most residency Program Directors will sincerely try to approach each candidate as a whole, placing less emphasis on standardized tests. Any program worth your time will understand that your Step or COMLEX score does not necessarily determine your ability to perform as a resident. This enlightened attitude is spreading within the world of GME, so take heart!

That being said, board exams are still needed because they help you to demonstrate that you've worked hard enough in school to build (and use) a strong framework of medical knowledge. We should view them as a hurdle to overcome, but not an assessment of our self-worth. It's just another standardized test that you have to conquer in order to earn the right to take care of patients.

With our rant out of the way, let's think about the pillars of board preparation:

1) a **comprehensive resource** for review
2) boards-style practice questions from third-party **Qbanks**
3) officially-sanctioned **simulated exams** (e.g., NBME and COMSAE exams).

Why these three? The comprehensive resource (like First Aid, Boards and Beyond, Lecturio, or Doctors in Training) will help you to review all of the most important material from your classes. The Qbanks (like UWORLD or Amboss) will help you to reinforce that material and apply your knowledge. The simulated exams will improve your test-taking endurance and will give you questions from the perspective of the actual test-writers (i.e., NBME and COMSAE exams come straight from the horse's mouth).

> *Note from Chase: "If I were to do one thing differently, it would NOT be selecting different study materials, using a greater variety of resources, or dedicating more hours per day to studying for the boards. It would be: 1) learning how to learn before the coursework becomes too intense, and 2) mastering one resource before moving onto another. Making low-yield flashcards and study materials wasted months of my time. And mastering one C-Rated resource is better than skimming ten A-Rated books."*

Next, you need to consider when you should begin preparing. For most students, this ranges from **2-8 months ahead of time**. Anecdotally, 3-4 months seems to be a fair average for students attending U.S. medical schools and 6-8 months for Caribbean and international medical schools.

When you feel ready to start studying for the boards, begin by picking your comprehensive resource(s) and a question bank. Quantify the amount of information (questions, pages, modules, and videos) you have to cover in the time available before your test and figure out how much studying you'll need to do per day.

For instance, you could start by reading 10 pages from a review book (and/or watching a couple of review videos) plus answering 10 practice questions per day. Plan to give each of these tasks 100% of your focus for deep learning.

Reading pages and watching videos are pretty straightforward tasks. But practice questions are *less-so*. Depending on your comfort level, you could do a random set of questions or subject-specific questions. But how much time will it take to answer 10 questions? Probably an hour! Why so much time? You will spend 10-20 minutes answering them, and then another 40-50 minutes reviewing the explanations.

To properly review a boards-style practice question, you should plan to **thoroughly read the ENTIRE explanation**, for both the correct answer choice and the incorrect answers. Then, you need to **identify any errors of thought**. (A description of Error Analysis will be provided in the next section.) Then, you should **highlight any new or unfamiliar terms** for future study. Consider putting these terms in a journal or flashcard deck for later review. As you advance in your studies, you will start to use more time for practice questions and less time creating new study materials. Finally, you will need to **update your existing study materials as needed** (like an Anki flashcard deck, a journal, or your comprehensive resource like First Aid).

One way to take your studying to the next level is to use the **Cover the Answers Method**. Cover the answer choices with an opaque card while reading the vignette. Then, after finishing the vignette, anticipate the correct answer *before* looking at your choices. Hopefully, your best guess will match one of the options. Test writers are instructed to craft ALL of their questions in a manner that will satisfy the "cover the answers test." This type of practice - though more time-consuming and mentally taxing - is a great way to identify knowledge gaps and to prevent the Illusion of Competence.

So, if you haven't picked up on this yet, it is crucial for you to answer and review MANY practice questions when preparing for the boards, usually somewhere between **2,000 to 7,000**. It takes months to get all of this done. Along the way, you'll pass through two general phases. The first phase is all about **maximizing accuracy**. Until the last couple of weeks before your board exam, you should focus on learning *as much as you can* to get the right answers (i.e., maximizing accuracy). This is the time when you should plan to spend about an hour for every 10 questions. Also, keep in mind that during this phase you are still being barraged with new information from your classes. You are both learning new material and reviewing old material, so it needs to be spread out over months of time to be effective.

The second phase is all about **maximizing endurance**. In the final weeks before your test, complete longer and longer question sets to maximize your endurance for test day. For reference, the USMLE Step 1 consists of ~280 questions spread over 8 hours, while the COMLEX Level 1 has ~400 questions spread over 9 hours. Both tests are comprehensive and exhausting. The endurance phase is also where those NBME and COMSAE exams come in; they are half-length practice tests that come straight from the test-writers, so you should plan to complete several of them. Track your progress during the endurance phase by spreading out your official practice tests over time. See an example below.

Weeks 1-3	Week 4	Weeks 5-7	Week 8	Weeks 9-11	Week 12
2 Hour Test (80 PQ) once per week	Rest	4 Hour Test (160 PQ) once per week	Rest	8 Hour Test (360 PQ) once per week	Exam Day

Once you are able to complete 4-5 hours in one sitting, feel free to test the waters by jumping into a full-length, eight-hour simulation. The whole point of this simulation is to mimic the test conditions as closely as possible. You will use the NBME or COMSAE testing software, follow their rules for breaks, put your phone away, pack a lunch, etc. This will give you a very realistic picture of your cognitive stamina leading up to the exam.

If you *really* want your practice simulations to be like the real deal, consider using a laminated printout of the Board Exam Grid that will be used at the testing center (see an example in the Appendix). You can use this as scratch paper for calculations during the test or to unload some of your crammed facts before starting the test. For example, many students will memorize a few acronyms and equations to place on the scratch paper.

You should also consider experimenting with all of the testing features available on the NBME and COMSAE software. These include the highlighter, strikethrough, marking for later review, and note-taking features. Many students opt not to use these features because they take up extra time, but if you practice with them beforehand in a low-stakes environment, it'll be easier to take advantage of them on test day.

To further enhance your test performance, you could also consider adding stress to your practice tests. For example, attempting to take a full-length, simulated exam in a noisy coffee shop, or manually reducing your time limit by 10-20 minutes. Why do this? Because if you can do this and stay focused during your practice, then nothing will rattle you on test day!

One final point to close out this section is focusing your attention on weak points. While it would be great to shore up *all* of your weaknesses, when you are coming to the end of your dedicated prep period, you will need to prioritize. If you are scoring 30% on physiology and 80% on microbiology within your Qbank, you obviously need to focus on physiology. But what if you are scoring 65% on psychology and 68% on pharmacology?

We have a solution for this kind of dilemma, which is based on **weighted averages**. Similar to a weighted GPA, you can mathematically estimate the relative importance of each subject on the boards. Thanks to the test breakdowns given by the NBME content outline and the NBOME Blueprint we can, for instance, see that Social Sciences (including Psychology) constitutes 1-5% of the exam, while Pharmacology is dispersed across 15-20% of the questions. So, even though you are scoring a little higher in pharmacology, it still makes more sense to focus on your pharmacology weaknesses than your psychology weaknesses. Though only a *guestimation*, we can use the following formula to assess the relative importance of our weighted subject matter:

Potential Gains =
Change in % of Subject Score x Total Discipline % of Exam

So, in the example given, let's assume that we want to assess what total difference we can expect on our exam score by bringing our current subject scores to 75%. That is taking Social Sciences from 65% to 75% and Pharmacology from 68% to 75%.

> Social Sciences: 10% (difference from 65% to 75%) x 5% (upper level is 5% of exam) = .005 or 0.5%. The maximum difference we can expect to gain is one-half of one percentage point.

> vs.

> Pharmacology: 7% (difference from 68% to 75%) x 20% (upper level is 20% of exam) = .014 or 1.4%.

So, in this example, the expected gains are ~3x higher if we were to focus on Pharmacology rather than Psychology! This isn't a difficult concept, but most students do not think of the board exams explicitly in these terms. Consider using this strategy to see where you can expect the greatest gains for your time and effort.

Becoming a Better Test-taker

How do you read a test question? No joke, think about this for a minute. More than likely, whatever strategy you have previously used will not be optimal for board exams. As mentioned above, this is a completely different test than most other standardized tests. If you have not yet looked at any board-style questions, this may be difficult to understand. You can find a booklet of practice examples and other related information on the USMLE Practice Materials page or the NBOME Practice & Preparation page.

The most commonly recommended strategy is to start with the question you are trying to answer, which is the last line in the question (the **interrogatory**). This provides two benefits. First, this uses the Priming Effect to bring your focused attention towards certain key phrases when reading the entire **vignette**. Second, this prevents you from losing time with pseudo-questions, which are questions that do not require any information in the clinical vignette to answer. Here's an example of a pseudo-question:

> A 74-year-old female presents to the office with complaints of chest pain, palpitations, and lightheadedness that started suddenly 30 minutes ago. She describes it as "crushing" pain. She has a ten-year history of poorly-controlled hypertension and hypercholesterolemia. Her father died of a myocardial infarction at age 64. Vital signs are significant for heart rate of 110 and blood pressure of 142/90. On exam, she is anxious appearing, sweating, and frequently clutching at her chest. EKG reveals ST elevations in leads AVL and V2-V5. What is the mechanism underlying myocyte damage during a myocardial infarction?

If you have not started medical training yet, this is a case of a patient who is having a heart attack (or myocardial infarction), given her presentation and risk factors for heart disease. But, if you looked at the interrogatory first, then you'd notice that it simply asks about the way in which heart cells are damaged by myocardial infarction. That's it. Did we need the patient's history? Did we need her family history or risk factors? Do we even need a patient to answer this question?! No. A better interrogatory for this question would look something like:

> Which of the following best describes the mechanism of injury caused by her underlying disease?

Though not frequently seen, you will run into a few pseudo-questions during your personal studies and on the boards. The Gold Book expressly forbids them, but some still slip through the cracks. It's very frustrating to waste precious time reading the vignette, just to get to the end and realize that all the preceding information was unnecessary to answer the interrogatory. Hence, we advise you to quickly peek at the interrogatory before reading the vignette.

From here, some suggest reading the answer choices next, while others advise against it. Really, where you go next depends on your personal preference. For some of us, it can be difficult to keep all the facts of the vignette straight without first looking at the answer choices. But others are unduly biased by looking at the answer choices and would rather wait to look at them until they've read the vignette and have come up with a potential solution on their own. Either way, for the vast majority of questions, you will need to read the entire question to come up with the right answer.

Over the last decade, the clinical vignettes (or question stems) on the boards have become more complex, longer, and more taxing on the student's working memory. You just won't see simple one- or two-liners these days. They must paint a picture for you and provide all the relevant information needed to answer the question. However, seeing the underlying pattern that is hidden within the monotonous wall of text is a challenging task. Here are some factors/tips that you should consider when approaching any vignette

Site of Care: Are we in the ED, the hospital, the operating room, or an ambulatory (outpatient) clinic? Considering the site of care will help you to determine the situation's urgency, the timing (i.e., acute or chronic), and it will hint at the types of diagnoses you should be thinking about. For example, you should not expect to see an exsanguinating patient at an ambulatory clinic; you would expect them to be hospitalized, in the OR, or presenting to the ED.

Demographics: Age, gender, race, culture, sexual activity, etc. will all predispose to certain disease processes that you'll learn about in medical school. Board exams will usually have the patient's demographics fit with the classic presentation of the disease. For example, a 4-year-old Norwegian boy with recurrent respiratory infections and "salty sweat" likely has cystic fibrosis.

Key Factors: There will be many extraneous details in any given vignette, but after being primed with the interrogatory, try to find the 3 key pieces of information to answer that question. It may be a piece of personal medical history, family history, lab tests, vital signs, severity of symptoms, acute vs. chronic, a classic "buzzword," or anything else in the stem. To keep track of these key factors, you have the ability to highlight on the exam; we recommend using this tool.

Eliminate the Clutter: The testing software will also allow you to strikethrough (or cross out) answer choices that you have ruled out. It takes very little time to do this, but it can help to streamline your thinking by removing distractions.

Make a choice: In the end, you have to pick an answer. If you don't know or are stuck between two answers and the seconds are ticking away, just go with your first impression and keep moving. You do not lose more points for guessing. Later in Part 2, we also give you a Tie-breaker Method that you can use (if there's enough time). Many students have heard the advice that, in general, switching your answer is a bad idea, but this isn't necessarily true. Most third-party question banks have a feature that analyzes how many questions were changed (and whether this change produced a correct or incorrect answer). Look at these analyses to see whether you tend to switch to the correct or incorrect answer.

Double Check: Always look at the interrogatory one last time after you have made an answer selection. It is very easy and very common to get lost in the information-dense vignette and to forget or misinterpret the actual question you need to answer.

The patient demographics, site of care, and chief complaint are usually provided in the first sentence of the question stem. One recommendation is to try to visualize a patient that fits this demographic and the environment where their care is being provided. Adding this kind of context in your mind's eye can be very helpful. You may even begin to develop certain avatars or mental models of specific patients and diseases. But while this strategy is very useful for taking standardized exams, its utility in real life is less significant. In clinical medicine, truly "classic" presentations are surprisingly uncommon.

When reading through a very long clinical vignette, you may find yourself confused, overwhelmed, and discouraged because you lost the storyline. Cognitive scientists have found that our working (short-term) memory can, on average, store 3 to 9 items during any given task [2]. There is some debate about the exact numbers and how widely this rule applies, but it is illustrative for our purposes. When working through a test question, most of us can only keep track of 3 to 9 variables from the vignette. But a lengthy vignette will have dozens of details that you need to sift through. If you have trouble keeping track of the data in your head, simply use the highlighter function and strikethrough tool to reduce cognitive load.

If you have used all your skills/tricks and still cannot come up with the right answer, mark the question for later. Just be sure to select your best guess before moving on. When revisiting a question that was overwhelming, make sure to break it down by pieces. Read one sentence at a time and think "Why did they give me this *specific* piece of information?" Though it may seem agonizing to spend 15+ seconds per line, deciphering through each variable of the question should help to present a single *best* answer choice. But only use this strategy if you have already answered *all* the other questions in the block. Time is precious on the boards.

One last point: accept that you won't know all the answers. Yes, you were probably one of the smartest kids growing up, but there's just too much information for any single person to know off the top of their head. Humbly accepting your limitations will save you a lot of grief on the boards and wards.

Conquering the Worm

"Great things come out of being hungry and cold.
Once you're pampered, you get lazy."
Rob Zombie

To overcome all the hurdles along our board exam journey, we must plan to work within their set of rules and to circumvent the common pitfalls that have been identified by previous test-takers. With this next section we are going to take you behind the curtain, inside the mind of a question writer.

For the purposes of this discussion, we will focus on the principles laid out by the NBME Gold Book [3], as the USMLE is the common exam taken by both MD and DO students. For the die-hard osteopaths out there, you don't need to worry because the NBOME uses very similar guidelines to craft the COMLEX.

Exam writers have a set of rules they are supposed to follow when writing a question. Knowing these rules allows us to assess what *they* are focusing on and, by extension, what they want *us* to focus on. According to the NBME Gold Book, the rules are as follows:

Rule 1: Each item should focus on an important concept or testing point.

Rule 2: Each item should assess the application of knowledge, not recall of an isolated fact.

Rule 3: The item lead-in should be focused, closed, and clear; the test-taker should be able to answer the item based on the stem and lead-in interrogatory alone.

Rule 4: All options should be homogeneous and plausible, to avoid cueing to the correct option.

Rule 5: Always review items to identify and remove technical flaws that add irrelevant difficulty or benefit savvy test-takers.

An acceptable board exam question must have a *single best answer*. Period. The best answer must have these qualities: 1) Be unambiguous and avoid imprecise language; 2) The lead-in question should be "closed" so that a test-taker can use the "cover-the-options" rule; 3) Question options can be judged as entirely true or entirely false on a single dimension; and 4) Incorrect answers can be partially or fully incorrect. We feel a 5th should be added here: patients *always* tell the truth (on the boards).

So, despite what we may think at times, board exam questions should never be made to "trick" us or to have two equally correct answer choices. However, if the question is testing a particularly nuanced point, then there may appear to be multiple correct answers. These rules, unfortunately, do not apply to third-party question bank companies. Though they try, most companies cannot dedicate sufficient resources to properly vet *all* of their questions to the extent that the NBME does. This is not a condemnation, but a note to be aware of and hopefully prevent frustration when using third-party resources.

Now let's look at these best-design qualities in practice. Fair warning, if you are reading this section as a pre-med, you may not be familiar with the specific content of these examples. However, you will be able to walk away with the key principles that will serve you well in medical school and beyond. See our first example below:

> A 20-year-old female presents to her physician's office with complaints of fatigue and an enlarging rash on her lower leg. She went hiking with her college ecology course two weeks ago. On exam, the rash is erythematous with central clearing. Which of the following microorganisms is most likely responsible for this patient's presentation?
>
> a) *S. aureus*
> b) *S. pyogenes*

c) *R. rickettsii*
d) *B. burgdorferi*
e) *T. pallidum*

Even without seeing a list of answer choices, this oversimplified vignette gives us the classic story for early Lyme disease. The patient 1) was hiking outside (suggesting an exposure to ticks), 2) presents with fatigue and rash, and 3) the rash has the classic "targetoid" shape of erythema migrans. Board exam questions can vary in length and complexity but should guide you towards one "best" diagnosis.

The previous question focused on the diagnosis of Lyme disease, based on the patient's history and physical exam. But, once you identified the underlying diagnosis, you needed to take it one step further to get the correct answer - you needed to know that Lyme disease is caused by the spirochete known as *Borrelia burgdorferi*. This was a simple second-order question that you can expect to see in abundance on the boards. Now, let's look at a similar example that is a little more complicated.

A 7-year-old boy presents to his physician's office with complaints of fatigue and a rash. He recently returned from a camping trip with his youth scouts organization. The rash is erythematous with a central clearing. What is the best choice of pharmacologic management for this patient?

a) Doxycycline
b) Gentamycin
c) Amoxicillin
d) Ceftriaxone
e) Azithromycin

Again, the question is written in a manner that can be answered before looking at the answer options. However, the interrogatory is different (best drug choice) and the demographic data are different (his age). Both of these are important to get the right answer. We have to know the underlying diagnosis (early Lyme disease) and the treatment, based on age and side-effect profile. Traditionally, doxycycline has been used to treat early Lyme disease in adults, but in children less than 8 years, doxycycline is not the preferred drug because it is known to stain permanent teeth. Instead, most physicians opt for an agent like amoxicillin, and this fun factoid provided great test fodder for the boards. (However, more recent studies have shown that doxycycline is probably still safe for children under 8 [4].)

Regardless of the details of this case, you can see how complicated a boards-style question can become. It takes time, effort, and repeated exposure for this kind of information to stick.

One quick principle we can take away from this example is to notice that, whenever a child is involved, you will need to think about how their management is different from that of a healthy adult. Kids should *not* be treated just like little adults. As you complete more practice questions, you'll start to pick up on these trends.

By definition, the exam writers should not throw in "trick questions," make them irrelevantly difficult or otherwise make the question unfair to a test-taker. We can assure you that every question on the boards is accurate and fair at the time of its writing (though the medical literature is constantly being updated). Each item is critically reviewed by an entire team of medical professionals and scientists. So, rather than pointlessly bucking against the system, you ought to develop a strategy to minimize errors and maximize your score.

Basic Exam Technique and Common Errors

Through our collective experiences, education, and expertise in medicine and academics, we have developed a few simple strategies that students can use when facing difficult test questions. Collectively, we refer to these tools as the **MedEdge Method**. Our approach has three essential elements: the **Basic Exam Technique,** the **Tie-breaker Technique,** and the **Post-Exam Autopsy**.

Basic Exam Technique

Step 1: If you 100% know the answer, choose it and move on... Not too complicated.

Step 2: Strike-out all known incorrect answers to reduce Cognitive Load.

Step 3: **Highlight** the Key Features, which are the 3 +/- 1 most important points in the vignette.

Step 4: **Rank** your preferred answers choices from 1-3. You may have multiples of each ranking (ex: Two choices that you mark with #1). Anything after #3, you should discard.

Step 5: Look for anything that could possibly be wrong with each of your remaining choices. **Partial False equals False.**

Step 6: **Re-read** the interrogatory and if your top choice is still #1, then choose it and move on.

Step 7: If you have more than a single #1, use the **Tie-breaker Technique** (see next section).

Although there are multiple steps above, you can complete all of them in a matter of seconds. Most students already do something like this in their head, but if you're really struggling with a question, we would recommend you externalize your thinking by highlighting, striking through, and listing out your top choices. Eventually, the process becomes automated. Let's use a sample question to practice the Basic Exam Technique. For this question, skip over Step 1 so you can go through the full exercise.

A 26-year-old woman presents to her doctor's office due to concerns of infertility. She has been unable to conceive for over a year despite discontinuing oral contraceptive pills. Menses occur at regular 28-day intervals. Her past history is significant for an episode of pelvic pain and vaginal discharge two years ago, which resolved without treatment. Pelvic exam showed no abnormalities. Her husband was assessed for infertility, but his workup showed no abnormalities. Which of the following is the most likely cause of this patient's infertility?

a) Premature ovarian failure
b) Insulin resistance
c) Ectopic endometrial tissue
d) Side effect of oral contraceptive pills
e) Fallopian tube damage

Step 1: If you 100% know the answer, choose it and move on.
Step 2: Strike-out all known incorrect options.
Step 3: Highlight key features: 1) infertile > one year, 2) menses normal, 3) remote history of pelvic pain and discharge
Step 4: Ranking.

*Below we provide some context for this question, then we illustrate the process with a helpful table and text.

Context:
   -Premature ovarian failure is the cessation of menses for 12+ months earlier than age 40 (i.e., early menopause)
   -Insulin resistance is commonly seen in polycystic ovarian syndrome (PCOS), which can predispose to fertility issues.
   -Ectopic endometrial tissue describes endometriosis, which can predispose to fertility issues.
   -OCPs use a combination of progesterone and estrogen to disrupt ovulation cycles and thereby prevent pregnancy. They

cause a host of side effects.

-Fallopian tubes may be damaged by physical insult, tumors, infectious diseases, and other causes. Damage to the tubes would predispose to infertility.

Basic Exam Technique in a Table

	Answer Choice	Rank	Reasoning
A	~~Premature Ovarian Failure~~	-	This patient has normal menses, not anovulation for >12 months
B	~~Insulin resistance~~	-	She does not display any of the other signs of PCOS (hirsutism, anovulatory cycles, etc.)
C	~~Ectopic endometrial tissue~~	-	She does not endorse the monthly/cyclic pain characteristic of endometriosis.
D	Side effect of oral contraceptive pills	2	She was taking OCPs before this issue started. Because I don't know ALL of the side effects of OCP's, I should consider this as a possibility. I'll mark it as a "2" for now.
E	Fallopian tube damage	1	Her remote history of pelvic pain and discharge is suspicious for pelvic inflammatory disease, which can cause damage/scarring of the fallopian tubes (producing infertility). This seems like the best answer.

Step 5: We did not have any answer choices that were clearly Partial False.

Step 6: Re-read the interrogatory, "Which of the following is the most likely cause of this patient's infertility?" Does our top choice *fully* answer this question? Yes, so we will plan to move on.

Step 7: A Tie-breaker was not needed for this question.

Note from Chase: In order to know the answer to most

questions on the boards, you need to be able to answer the question, "What is the underlying diagnosis?" Try getting into the habit of answering this for every question, even if that is not the final interrogatory you are prompted with. Questions on workup, treatments, and mechanisms will all revolve around the suspected diagnosis.

In this example, we are able to limit the likely options down to two. We may not have all of the facts, which is quite common, but with the right strategy it is usually possible to whittle down to the 2-3 most likely options. Keep the Key Features in mind and always try to find those pesky Partial False answers.

When studying for the exam, it will be supremely helpful to **keep a record** of your rationale on any particularly difficult questions. This gives you the opportunity to find your bad habits and correct them ahead of time. It will also help you to identify knowledge gaps. These notes will help to form the basis for any Post-exam Autopsy that you perform in your dedicated study time (see next section).

When using third-party question banks, any test-taking error is simply reported as "Incorrect," but it cannot identify *why* you missed the question. Was it a silly misread, a knowledge gap, time-pressure, or a significant cognitive error? Additionally, specific knowledge gaps are almost impossible to detect through Qbank reports and statistics, because they only report on broad categories like your performance on questions related to Cardiology or Statistics. While this information is helpful early-on in directing your studies, in the final weeks of test prep you need to micro-target your individual weaknesses. Hence, we recommend that you keep your own record.

Back to the example we used above, you may have noticed that we did not need to use Steps 5 or 7, and Step 6 was very straightforward. This will not always be the case, so it is a good idea to consistently use ALL of the steps when you encounter a tricky question (if you plan to use our Basic Exam Technique). Harkening back to our section on Habits, *perfect practice makes perfect performance*. Now, let's run the scenario again, but we will assume that you didn't actually know the answer.

Answer Choice		Reasoning
A	Premature Ovarian Failure	?	I didn't know what age met POF criteria, but 26 seems *pretty* early.
B	Insulin Resistance	-	I didn't make the connection between this answer option and PCOS.
C	Ectopic endometrial tissue	?	I didn't understand that this described endometriosis.
D	Side effect of oral contraceptive pills	?	I didn't know the any of the side effects of OCPs.
E	Fallopian tube damage	?	I wasn't sure of the causes of fallopian tube damage, but knew this could cause infertility.

Here, we can see that there is a potential for a tie-breaker between A, C, D, and E. However, we still knew enough to suspect that E was the best contender. In this case, *choose the strong hunch over the complete guess*. Based on the example above, our analysis of this question would suggest that we need to more thoroughly study several topics in OBGYN, particularly the diagnostic criteria of premature ovarian failure, the features of PCOS, the presentation of endometriosis, and the side effect profile of OCPs. All of these would be great additions to a study journal.

You can find a condensed version of the Basic Exam Technique in the Appendix, or download a copy by visiting FreeMedEd.org/MedStudent. At this point, we suggest that you put down our book and go try out a few practice questions before you return. Practice the basics a few times, perhaps using an online quiz like the University of Utah's free WebPath quizzes. You won't get much out of reading this book unless you put in the work.

Okay, now that you're back... Below you will find our **Error Analysis** table, which lists out common errors that test-takers make, why the error happens, and ways to correct the mistake. There's certainly some overlap between categories and multiple errors can be made on a single question, but breaking things down like this will help to demystify what we mean by performing a Post-exam Autopsy. It may feel overwhelming to use a table like this after each exam, but most of the ideas are completely intuitive, so it'll become second-nature with a little bit of practice.

ERROR	CONCEPT	CORRECTION
1. Negligence Errors		
1a. Misreads	Misread/misunderstood the interrogatory, key features, or answer options.	Slow down when reading interrogatory and stem. Pause after each sentence to assess understanding. Use Highlighting and Strikethrough tools to reduce cognitive load.
1b. Impulse Control	Allowed distracting facts or answer choices to bias your decision making. Jumping to conclusions, or blocking out reasonable options.	Stay neutral until you read the entire stem. Remind yourself of the pernicious effects of Recency Bias, the Availability Heuristic, and other cognitive biases during your practice tests.
1c. Honing Miss	Failed to locate the 3 +/- 1 most important Key Features the test writer wanted you to notice.	Consider: is this a Knowledge Gap or Misread? Did you favor a supportive feature over a Key Feature?
2. Test Procedure Errors		
2a. Stamina & Time Management (Endurance)	Spending too much time on a minority of questions within a block. Missing more questions in later blocks.	If spending >70 sec on a question, put your best guess, mark it and move on! Build up stamina by taking longer and longer tests (up to 400 PQ). Plan for longer breaks before the later blocks (if able).
2b. Double-Check	Failing to re-read the interrogatory after making your answer choice. Failing to mark/flag and double-check difficult questions.	Treat this like a bad habit. Consider implementing a reward system and decreasing your reward for each slip-up. Keep track of your errors with a record*

2c. Tie Breakers	Failing to implement proper exam technique and a tie-breaker technique (discussed next).	If not due to a Knowledge Gap, consider where the failure took place. Make sure to properly use highlighting and strikethrough. Reassess Key Features and re-read the interrogatory before committing to your answer.
3. Conceptual/Study Errors		
3a. Knowledge Application Miss	Failure to apply current knowledge correctly.	Focus your next practice session on material related to this concept. Draw it out, write it out, talk it out, or explain it to a peer.
**3b. Knowledge Gap	Never heard of or learned about the information being tested.	Thoroughly read the explanation. Mark the topic for later review. Add this to your study materials for future retrieval practice.

*See the Appendix for a sample Error Monitoring schedule.
**You can also subdivide Knowledge Gap Errors into Diagnosis errors, Procedure errors, Medication/Treatment errors, etc. to narrow your focus for future studies.

Tie-breaker Technique and Post-Exam Autopsy

You've already taken plenty of exams in your academic career. So, it's no surprise that - just like in undergrad - the multiple-choice tests you encounter in medical school will have questions that force you to pick between two or more plausible answers. How can you reliably pick the best option? Below is a four-step process that can help you to make a rational choice about how to break the tie. The **Tie-breaker Technique** should only be used for questions that you have marked for later review (after you have selected an answer for each question in the block). It will take time to work through the steps, so you need to save this for the end. The clock is working against you on test day!

Tie-breaker Technique

Step 1: Re-read the entire vignette, then review the highlighted Key Features. Consider where your thinking might have gone astray.

Step 2: Make a brief Pro-Con list to assess the strengths and weaknesses of each of your top choices.

Step 3: Re-prime yourself with only the top choices in mind and then re-read the interrogatory. Which option *best* answers the question?

Step 4: If you still haven't identified a *single* best answer, go with your first instinct.

At the end of Steps 1-3, if you still have no clue about the correct answer, then this is likely a Category 3 error and related to some type of knowledge gap. If you have no new thoughts or information to sway your decision, and the Pro-Con list did not help, then going with your first instinct is probably your best option. If you end up getting the question wrong due to a Category 3 error, then you know where to focus your future studies. No need to panic.

Now that we have covered the Basic Exam Technique and the Tie-breaker Technique, we have arrived at the last step of the MedEdge Method: the **Post-exam Autopsy**.

Third party Qbanks perform a basic Post-exam Autopsy for you by identifying incorrect answers, breaking them down by subject area, and recording whether you switched from correct to incorrect (or vice versa). However, an important limitation of these programs is their inability to describe HOW you arrived at the wrong answer. Was it a knowledge gap? Misapplication of existing knowledge? Were you crunched for time? There's no substitute for replaying your thought process to figure out where you went astray.

Benefit your future studies by incorporating your incorrect questions into your study notes, flashcard deck, and/or exam journal. When making flashcards, it is important to write out the question in your own words. Do not copy-paste the entire vignette onto the front of the card. Instead, word a question that focuses on the main topic(s) missed and summarize the explanation on the back of the card. By translating it into your own words, you are required to synthesize the material, which is thought to promote deeper learning [5].

Drawing inspiration from Deliberate Practice, if you truly want to get better, it is essential to scrutinize your mistakes. In the Post-exam Autopsy, you will identify your errors of thought, face up to your lucky guesses, and log your weak points (see our sample log in the Appendix). Whenever possible, we recommend going through this exercise. One way to keep yourself organized for the Post-exam Autopsy is to keep a copy of our Error Analysis table on-hand (see in previous section).

If you're stuck or unsure of what to do with all this information, consider bringing your Post-exam Autopsy to a trusted friend, teacher, tutor, or mentor. You can also reach out through our FreeMedEd social media pages and see if the community can be of assistance. See a full list of these pages at the end of Part 4.

Final Test Day Tips

Any thorough test prep chapter must also include tips and suggestions for Exam Day. All of the information needed for showing up on time and what to bring (or not bring) can be found on the Prometric Testing Center site, the USMLE Testing Bulletin, or the NBOME website. These rules may change from time to time, so it is best to get the information *straight from the source.*

At this point, you have read our suggestions for nutrition, sleep, and physical activity in Part 1. There are no special changes required for test day if you have been healthy and active leading up to it, so there is little to add here. Keep everything as you would on your healthiest days, and maintain this schedule for at least a week before the exam.

No matter how hard you train physically or mentally, there is always a chance for something to go wrong. Whether it be your computer not working, cognitive fatigue setting in early, a noisy test-taker next to you, or a string of very difficult questions that throw off your entire block. In Part 1, you saw how to improve your Mindset and Resilience, making it easier to shrug off these events. At a minimum, when your stress level is high, simply take 10 seconds to sit back in your chair and close your eyes. A few deep, cleansing breaths can do wonders, and you only used 10 seconds of an eight-hour exam. Notice we said "used" and not "wasted." Stay positive!

Another tip that we mentioned previously is to use the laminated grid paper you are given before the exam to reduce Cognitive Load. We provided a realistic rendering of this paper in the Appendix. There are many techniques that can be used, so figure out what works best for you ahead of time. You can use both sides of the paper during the exam, but you are warned not to erase anything on it. Take this into consideration when determining the quantity and size of the content you add. Below are some tips for how to use the laminated grid paper:

1) Use the grid paper as a mental "dumping ground" at the beginning of your exam. Unload any mnemonics, difficult

topics, or math equations so you don't have to remember them later.

2) Use it solely to perform calculations.

3) Use it as a space to conduct parts of our Basic Exam Technique or Tie-breaker Technique (or to write out the steps of these procedures).

4) If you are artistic, you may consider drawing graphic representations that you have prepared for the exam, or even Visual Markers you've created while preparing for the boards (see Part 3 for more details about mnemonics). The less you have to remember under stress, the better. Also, these sketches don't need to be works of art, so long as *you* know what they mean. You are the only person who will see them.

Closing Thoughts - Part 2

Put these tips into practice right away. Our tools, such as the Basic Exam Technique or the Tie-breaker Technique, may seem a little complicated at first, but with practice they will become second-nature.

Eventually, there will be a point of diminishing returns for your book studies. If available, try to get some clinical time so you can see how all the theory is put into practice. Your school may not offer official clinical experiences until your 3rd and 4th year. However, there are often free clinics looking for volunteers.

Hospitals, emergency medical services, dialysis centers, and nursing homes may also provide options to shadow or gain hands-on experience. However, with your busy academic curriculum, it is advised that you be very selective with these outside opportunities. Only choose those that will specifically fill in your knowledge gaps and provide relevant experience.

In Part 3 of this book, we will explore the fascinating topic of accelerated learning strategies. Medical students these days are getting more exposure to accelerated learning through resources produced by third-party medical education companies like Sketchy Medical and Picmonic. However, few of us receive any formal instruction on how to use accelerated learning strategies. The next section will explore some of the basics and suggest ways to apply them.

References - Part 2

References can also be found at https://freemeded.org/book-references/

1. Burk-Rafel J et al. (2017) Study behaviors and USMLE Step 1 performance: Implications of a student self-directed parallel curriculum. URL: https://scholarrx.com/wp-content/uploads/2019/11/Burk-Rafel_RIME-Study-Behaviors-and-USMLE_AcadMed_2017-1.pdf

2. Saaty TL & Ozdemir MS (2003) Why the magic number seven plus or minus two? URL: https://www.sciencedirect.com/science/article/pii/S0895717703900835

3. NBME Gold Book. URL: https://www.nbme.org/learningportal/X_Resources/Multimedia/IWW-Gold-Book.pdf

4. Todd SR et al. (2015) No visible dental staining in children treated with doxycycline for suspected Rocky Mountain Spotted Fever. URL: https://www.jpeds.com/article/S0022-3476(15)00135-3/pdf?ext=.pdf

5. Hans DM. The effectiveness of paraphrasing strategy in increasing university students' reading comprehension and writing achievement. URL: https://pdfs.semanticscholar.org/6d03/f4606dab569ce13a638432cebde613e35649.pdf

PART 3: ACCELERATED LEARNING AND MNEMONICS

Introduction to Accelerated Learning

One of the most common requests we received on the Medical Mnemonist Podcast is for step-by-step instructions on how to apply accelerated learning strategies and memory techniques into one's personal studies. There is a lot of debate about some of the hyperbolic statements made by speed-reading instructors and other accelerated learning gurus. Few robust studies can back up their claims. However, just like any other self-help or personal development scheme, what matters most is that the participant "buys in" and puts in the effort to better themselves. Our overall experience with these tactics has been favorable, so we wanted to include them in the book for your benefit.

Okay, now that our disclaimer is out of the way... Did you know that every year there is a US Memory Championship? At this event, contestants will memorize the order of a deck of cards in seconds, recite thousands of randomly generated digits, and even memorize long poems verbatim after a single pass. These contests were popularized by the recently published book, *Moonwalking with Einstein,* written by Joshua Foer. Initially, his interest in the area of memory competitions was for purely *journalistic* reasons, but he soon found himself practicing for (and ultimately winning) the US Memory Championships. Foer proved the point that even an average person can benefit from accelerated learning techniques.

Supporting this notion, recent studies have utilized MRI [1] and functional MRI [2] evaluation of the brains of several memory champions and found that their brains were nothing special. While you can see structural differences in the hippocampus after weeks of

149

intensive memory training [2], there's no indication that memory champions were born with any innate advantages.

With proper training, we can ALL have better memories. We can remember people's names and faces better. We can remember our passwords, phone numbers, and account numbers better. And, of more immediate concern, we can better remember medical facts when they are needed on the boards and wards.

Speed Reading

"It's what you practice in private that you
will be rewarded for in public."
Tony Robbins

Pre-Test: On a scale of 1-7 (1 = never and 7 = always) rate these questions.

#	Question/Statement	SCORE
1	I skim the title, headings, and subheadings before reading the chapter.	/7
2	I read the chapter summary and vocabulary before reading the main text.	/7
3	I quickly read through the paragraph/page, pointing out important names, dates, places, and keywords that look relevant to the section.	/7
4	I read the section at a variable speed according to the complexity of the material.	/7
5	I recall the material at the end of every few paragraphs and again at the chapter's end.	/7
6	I purposely set aside training time to read irrelevant materials at a faster speed than I am comfortable.	/7
7	I monitor my reading skills for progress by journaling or otherwise keeping records.	/7
	TOTAL	/49

Did you know that Theodore Roosevelt was known to read three books a day when he wished? There are many historical accounts that he frequently read a book a day before breakfast. Was he superhuman? This is a commonly touted anecdote in the accelerated learning community. What is less frequently mentioned is that Jimmy Carter was also able to read at these speeds after he completed a speed-reading course [3].

So, first things first... eliminate any doubts about yourself. You can do it too, with some training. According to *The Key to Study Skills*, written by Drs. Lev and Anna Goldentouch, it takes about 8-12 weeks of dedicated practice (~30 minutes per day) to become proficient with most accelerated learning techniques [4]. Unfortunately, if you have already begun medical school, this can be hard to squeeze in, but we will try to provide a reasonable approach to doing so.

The SQ3R System

In the 1940's, an educator named Francis P. Robinson published the book, *Effective Study*, wherein he introduced the world to his system for reading comprehension known as **SQ3R**. His book can be found in the public domain if you'd like to read it, but we will summarize the main points here. SQ3R stands for **Survey, Question, Read, Recite,** and **Review**. Most speed-reading courses use some variant of Robinson's system. This technique is not, in and of itself, speed-reading. However, it provides the best framework to maximize comprehension while speed-reading.

The first step is to Survey the text. By taking just a few seconds to flip through the chapter, you will notice the section headings, keywords, dates, names, tables and figures. During the Survey stage, about 95-99% of the words are skipped (i.e., it's a cursory glance). This quick scan of the chapter harnesses the Priming Effect, which will help to ramp up your attention when you come across these key phrases later.

After the Survey stage - but before you formally Read - you should take up to 30 seconds to formulate the central Question(s) being considered by the text. If the text has a list of these questions somewhere in the chapter (or review questions at the end), you could check your Question(s) against the author's.

With your curiosity piqued, now is the time to formally Read the text in its entirety. While reading, you will come across the key names, dates, vocabulary, etc. that were noted in the Survey stage. Think about how/why those keywords stood out and how they help to answer the central Question(s). Actively reading and taking advantage of the Priming Effect in this way is thought to increase comprehension [5]. Also, by looking ahead with your Survey, you may have seen a figure or table that helps to summarize a long section of text. So, rather than struggling your way down a large wall of text (or re-reading), you could simply jump ahead to the table or figure to get the main points.

Another difference between SQ3R and standard reading (from

beginning to end) is the step where you Recite what you've read. At the end of a long paragraph and/or each page, actively recite the key points you gleaned from the text above. This harnesses the short-term benefits of Retrieval Practice (which we discussed previously). Retrieval practice is well-known to boost retention, so you don't feel like all the words are coming in through your eyes and then shooting out the back of your head. An alternative to *verbally* reciting the text is to create study materials as you go along, like a mind map (which can really super-charge your learning [6]). Mind maps and other visual aids will be discussed later in Part 3.

Finally, after you have done the steps of Survey, Question, Read, and Recite, it is time to do one final Review, where you recap the important points from the chapter. This review can be bolstered by answering any practice questions available to you, or by talking things out with a friend. Whenever explaining complex subjects like medical science, try to limit your use of jargon whenever possible. Not only will this help your studies, but it's a useful habit to get into for your future clinical practice. When a patient is sitting in front of you, you have to find a way to communicate in a manner they will understand.

> *Note from Chase: If this is totally new to you, it will take some time to get the hang of SQ3R. Even after months of trying to use this strategy, I still caught myself trying to rush through reading like I always had in the past. It is easy to fall back into what is "comfortable." Practicing mindfulness has helped me to course-correct when I start to slip back into bad habits.*

One last point: when trying to get into the habit of SQ3R reading, it may be helpful to **keep the steps written down on your bookmark** or to have another way of reminding yourself before you sit down to read.

Below is a brief summary of SQ3R for your benefit:

1) **Survey**: flip through the chapter to find the key words and phrases.

2) **Question**: identify the central question(s) answered by the text.
3) **Read**: actively read the text.
4) **Recite**: actively recite what you've learned while reading (verbally or otherwise).
5) **Review**: perform one final recap and recitation of the text. Answer any practice questions provided by the authors.

Pacers

Much of the speed-reading training nowadays is based on Evelyn Wood's work, which she popularized with the Reading Dynamics Institute. In fact, she is credited with coining the term "speed-reading." Her work was so popular in the 1950s and 60s that many presidents of the era required their staff to take her course, including presidents Kennedy, Nixon, and Carter. One of the techniques emphasized by Wood is the use of a pacer.

It's unfortunate, but many children attempt to read with their finger in grade school just to have this practice trained out of them. It's a simple hack that allows the reader to concentrate their attention. In the digital age, many of us have a hard time keeping our attention on the articles we read, so we end up skimming. But in medical school, you cannot skim the material and expect to pass. Using a pacer can improve both your focus and your reading speed [8]. A pacer can be anything the reader wishes - a finger, a mouse cursor, a pencil, a notecard, whatever!

This technique is useful, but only to a degree. If you want to achieve much faster speeds, you'll need to be open to trying less conventional approaches. It is much easier to watch a tutorial than to explain some of the different strategies in writing. But for the sake of completeness, let's cover some of the more common alternative pacing strategies. Most of these focus on different ways to physically look at the words on the page.

Start things off by picking up a book that you don't particularly care about. Your default reading pattern for the English language is to read from left-to-right, one line at a time. Using a pacing object can speed this up. But, if you want to try something different, then you can try changing the movement of the pacer and/or the pattern you use to scan across the page. This helps to prevent our normal tendency to backtrack on a page when we feel we have missed something. One easy way to limit re-reading is to place a **notecard** _above_ **the line** you're currently reading and simply move it down the text as you read, line-by-line (thus covering the preceding lines of text).

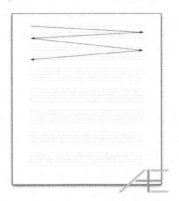

Next, the zig-zag pattern is probably the second most common. This requires the reader to widen their peripheral vision to take in multiple rows at a time. The pacing object will start on one line, moving left to right as before. However, when moving to a lower line, the finger moves at a diagonal from right to left, never lifting away from the page.

The target can start at the next line down, but many speed-readers will pick 2-4 lines down. Isn't this skipping huge chunks of the text? Not when combined with peripheral vision reading to take in all the keywords, as well as *backwards reading*. WHAT!? I can't read backwards! Though the concept sounds counterintuitive, if not impossible, you would be surprised how well your brain can adjust. In fact, you understand wacky sentences every time you watch Star Wars.

"Powerful you have become."

"Mourn them do not. Miss them do not."

"Much to learn, you still have, my young padawan."
Yoda

In most languages, including English, we are used to the subject-verb-object pattern. But Yoda doesn't speak this way. He uses an unusual object-subject-verb pattern. Despite its peculiarity, we can understand Yoda-speak. Further, because we generally read words as a whole, and not letters individually, the words themselves remain intact. This is one reason the zig-zag pattern is a feasible approach.

It is important to note that, when speed reading, we are not trying to take in every single word and retain every single fact. Depending on the type of text, only a small percentage may be required to understand its essential content.

If line-by-line is considered the first tier, and zig-zag a second tier, then the next stage is an adaptable third tier. We say *adaptable* because its use depends on the width of the text. A rough estimate is that the average number of words per line is usually around 12 (+/- 2) for fiction, closer to 16 for smaller font size, and more like 20+ for a school textbook. Obviously, there is great variation, but these will be used as examples for the last tier.

The third tier requires training the peripheral vision for reading, also called parafoveal vision. Yes, the fovea is the clearest part of our visual field. And yes, that requires us to look directly at an object for the clearest picture. But do we need the clearest vision to read a book? In theory, not really. In fact, parafoveal vision is proposed to decrease "foveal load" [9] and may decrease subsequent processing by areas of the brain related to the foveal vision field [10]. In other words, the written text seen by the area around our fovea may not be the clearest material, but it is adequate to decrease the workload of the foveal neurons and allow the brain to begin deciphering words in a wider field of view.

Do you know anyone, maybe yourself, who requires glasses or contact lenses for their vision? Have you ever lost them or forgotten them somewhere? Even with impaired vision, most of us can still make out street signs, certain texts, or even the number pad on our phone despite lacking our reading assistance devices. We are already familiar with the structure and shape of our native language, making it easier to decipher, even when it is unclear. Of course, this depends on many factors like our familiarity with the environment or the severity of our visual defects, but the principle holds true.

With all that being said, we hope that you're at least open to the idea that alternative scanning patterns are possible. If you want to try some of them for yourself, check out exercises like Visual Angle Training from the Key To Study website [11]. There are even some higher-level scanning strategies like the vertical S-shape and the straight line down the middle. We're not sure if this is a skill that

EVERYONE can develop, but there are enough reports to give it some credence.

Howard Berg has held the Guinness Book World Record for speed reading since 1987. In an interview, Mr. Berg stated that he can read approximately 80 pages per minute! [12] Luckily, most of us would be happy with just a hundred more words per minute. Even if you don't think the more extreme tiers are possible for you, the first two tiers are sufficient to increase the speed of many readers.

Subvocalization

What is subvocalizing? This is when we read some text and narrate it silently to ourselves. If you think about it, subvocalizing will limit your reading speed to the words-per-minute (WPM) of your internal monologue. If we consider using a pacing object to be the first *physical* step to speed reading, then silencing the internal voice is the first *mental* step. Note that these two changes are to be made simultaneously. Pacing while subvocalizing kind of defeats the purpose. The average person reads at a speed of around 150-250 WPM, and this happens to be the average rate of speech for most adults. Coincidence?

Unfortunately, as children we are all taught to read aloud to the class. We would read slowly and deliberately to avoid embarrassment. But we are never taught to break the habit when reading to ourselves, which ultimately slows down our reading speed. As adults, we have much more reading to do (and less time), so we ought to rid ourselves of this juvenile hang up.

So, now that we understand what subvocalization is and why it plagues many of us, what is there to do about it? There are a few decent options. Some say to chew gum or keep your tongue to the roof of your mouth when reading. Sometimes, just forcing yourself to read at a pace that's 50% faster than your baseline speed will silence your internal monologue. The Key To Study website recommends a tiered progression, which can be found on their Subvocalization Suppression Training page [13].

There is a bit of a learning curve, but it'll be worth the effort. Start with a single 10-15 minute session each day and see where it takes you.

Note from Chase: Sometimes concentrating on longer and deeper breaths while reading helps to suppress subvocalization. This hack came to me pretty naturally because I use deep breathing as a part of my meditation practice. And, for some reason, I think my comprehension has INCREASED by reading faster!

Bear in mind that, at times, subvocalization will return. This is normal and it's nothing to fret about. If anything, it's a sign of self-awareness. Simply re-initiate your strategy to suppress subvocalization (chew gum, increase pace, breathe, etc.) and keep moving down the page!

Saccadic Reading

Saccades are quick movements that our eyes make between fixed points when scanning across a field, like when our eyes are scrambling across a page to see each word. Technically, all reading is "saccadic reading," so this is more accurately termed "limited saccadic reading" or "limited fixation reading." What we may not realize is that we use an excessive number of saccades to get through a single line of text.

Speed reading sources say the human eye can take in around 12-15 characters, horizontally, per saccade. However, we experience many saccades per second [14]. What this means is that we are not being efficient with our reading, often due to back-reading (corrective saccades) or attempting to read each word instead of groups of words. To get around this, advanced speed readers form mental columns on a page.

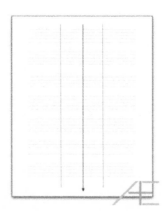

Depending on the reader's skill level and the number of words per line, forming 3 columns per page is a good start. Focus your eyes on the middle column and move down the page. While you're reading the middle column, your eyes will also take in the columns on either side of the middle column (as a part of your parafoveal vision). If, as in the Pacer section, you are wondering about decreased vision on the periphery, try this hypothetical scenario:

> *You are driving down an unfamiliar road. Suddenly, a stop sign pops out from its hiding place behind a tree. Immediately you hit the brakes, stopping just before you would have run the stop sign.*

Did you read the letters **S-T-O-P** on the sign? Probably not. You were able to recognize the word, sign shape, and color from previous experience. With some training, you can have a similar experience when reading. Even when reading at a normal speed, let's say 200 WPM, you are not always reading each and every word, especially when it comes to commonly used words. We can gloss over a few words or phrases and still ascertain the meaning of the sentence. Certain letters and words generally follow others, so there is a pattern we can take advantage of. In fact, the words don't even have to be spelled correctly. Psycholinguists have studied this phenomenon and produced sentences like this:

> "It deosn't mttaer waht oredr the ltteers in a wrod are in bcuseae the huamn mnid deos not raed ervey lteter by istlef, but the wrod as a wlohe."

Rearranging the letters of the words does not decrease the accuracy of your interpretation [15]. This is especially true for smaller words, when the first and last letter remain the same and when letter-transposition does not produce another real word. This is called the **Word Superiority Effect**, where whole words are visually processed faster than individual letters [16]. Thanks to the Primacy Effect and Recency Effect [17], the theory that we best remember the first and last objects in a grouping, we can simply focus more on the first and last letters in a string of letters (i.e., words) to decipher their meaning. However, some of this effect may be lost in your peripheral visual fields [18].

In practice, this means that - even when reading faster than your baseline WPM - you can still absorb the necessary information. Some studies have shown that harnessing saccadic reading can significantly increase the reading speed of an average person [19]. Others suggest that people who practice mental discipline, such as meditation, tend to perform better with saccadic reading training [20]. However, like many of the techniques explained in this book, they are not always natural at first. It is common to decrease in speed and comprehension initially until you become more comfortable with it.

If you struggle to visually place vertical lines down your pages at first, there are digital programs out there that can help, such as EyeCanLearn. Many browsers now have a Reading Mode (or other extensions) that help to limit distractions (i.e., advertisements) and to streamline your reading. Or you can begin to train your parafoveal vision and minimize your saccades per line the old-fashioned way: by simply drawing vertical lines down the page to make three columns. You can expect noticeable progress within a week or two of dedicated practice. Like any other new skill, the more time you put into it, the better your results will be.

Speed Training

If you have practiced the above techniques, and they are beginning to feel a little more natural, this section will provide more tips to boost your WPM. Obviously, you don't have thousands of hours to become a master speed reader like Dr. Lev Goldentouch who claims to read 1500 WPM at 85% retention, 5000 WPM at 20% retention, and 10,000 WPM at 10% retention [21]. You're looking for more modest gains.

The first step is to set realistic goals. Jumping from 200 WPM to 400 WPM in 3-6 weeks is a reasonable goal for most college-educated adults. Even if you only have 10-15 minutes available per day, commit that time to personal growth in this area. Reading faster has an amplifying effect on other skills in your life, particularly for studying and test-taking.

There are different schools of thought regarding speed training. Some suggest aiming for speed first, comprehension later. Others advocate the opposite approach. Regardless, here are two examples for readers starting at 200 WPM:

SPEED PATHWAY		COMPREHENSION PATHWAY	
Practice Speed (WPM)	Comprehension Goal (%)	Practice Speed (WPM)	Comprehension Goal (%)
200	200 (100%)	200	200 (100%)
400	200 (50%)	400	300 (90%)
600	300 (50%)	500	400 (85%)
800	400 (50%)	600	500 (80%)
1200	600 (50%)	700	600 (75%)

As you can see, in the Speed Pathway we are only aiming for 50% retention, so this type of training may not be best for medical students. Comprehension naturally rises with additional practice, but the Speed Pathway is meant more for speed reading competitors. In contrast, the Comprehension Pathway would be a better option for most medical students who need to retain what they read (ideally on the first go-around).

Setting the reading speed, or WPM, is easy with apps like Accelareader. Unfortunately, these kinds of apps have a hard time simultaneously training your parafoveal vision. In the end, it may be best to train by analog means: by dividing the text into three columns, counting up the words in the article, and setting a timer based on your WPM goal.

Initially, the training can be uncomfortable. You are pushing yourself to a greater reading speed than you are used to, which will temporarily reduce your comprehension, possibly to 30% or less [22]. This is fine. At first, it feels distressing to understand *even less* of what you are reading when trying to become a faster reader, but be consistent in your practice and you'll eventually get it.

One way to ease your anxiety about low comprehension is to practice speed training with unimportant/easy reading materials, like magazine articles or blog posts (or your uncle's most recent rant on social media). Grab a random book from your shelf or head to the public library.

For reference, the average book will have about 250-300 words per page. You can get an idea of words per page by multiplying the average number of lines per page X words per line. Let's assume it is 300 words per page; then finishing the page in 60 seconds means you are reading at 300 WPM. Read at this baseline pace for 5 minutes. Then, take a break and set a stopwatch to read each page in 45 seconds (450 WPM). Then slow down to 300 WPM again.

Similar to driving on a highway, when you acclimate to faster reading speeds, the slower speeds *feel* much slower and it feels like you have more time to digest the text. Use this kind of pattern to progressively increase your reading speed and have your progress be guided by a Comprehension Pathway. Gauging comprehension will always be more challenging than gauging WPM. In medical school, your comprehension is primarily determined by high-stakes exams, but you should plan to more regularly assess comprehension with practice tests from your textbooks and third-party Qbanks.

Organize What You've Read

Congratulations, you're a speed-reader, clocking in at >1000 WPM with >80% comprehension. Or, at the very least, you have seen modest improvements. This will save precious minutes each day, hours each week, and days each year.

Now you need to figure out what to do with all of the material you plan to read in the years to come. After all, increased reading speed doesn't really matter if you cannot remember (or reference) the material. Forgetting where you learned an intriguing fact can be very annoying.

You can easily save HTML documents or news articles with browser plug-ins like Pocket and InstaPaper. These apps also provide a distraction-free Reading Mode, and other nifty features, to make reading more efficient.

If you're reading research papers and need a place to keep them organized, then a citation manager like Mendeley, RefWorks, EndNote or Zotero can help you get the job done. All of these programs work nicely with Word and LibreOffice. Not only can you use them to organize your research and easily cite papers, they can help you to find related articles and to collaborate with colleagues.

In medical school, as well as later training, you will read countless articles and updates. Being able to reference these quickly will be helpful for your studies and your practice. Starting a cloud drive or Evernote and saving these documents early on is a great idea. Consider organizing by discipline, specialty, or disease. If an article belongs in multiple categories, copy it to each of the relevant folders.

But what about other resources outside of academic articles or webpages? Most digital readers have a highlighting feature, or you can copy/paste to your note-taking app of choice. The Kindle app even allows you to save notes and quotes from the material you are reading. Physical books are less flexible, but you can always type out your notes or take a snapshot of important pages to save for later. All of this stuff can easily become cluttered, so try to have an organization schema planned out ahead of time.

Memory Hacks & Techniques

"Memory is like a spiderweb that catches new information.
The more it catches, the bigger it grows.
And the bigger it grows, the more it catches."
Joshua Foer

Pre-Test: On a scale of 1-7 (1 = never and 7 = always) rate these questions.

#	Question/Statement	SCORE
1	I utilize visual images to help me remember complex or difficult material.	/7
2	I have a set time each day or week to train with these techniques (or I am comfortable with my current skill level).	/7
3	I have several techniques to help create images for difficult work or scientific jargon.	/7
4	I use spaced repetition with my visual mnemonics to solidify them in my memory.	/7
5	I keep notes or drawings as a backup for study material.	/7
6	I place my mnemonics in Linked pathways or Memory Palaces to keep them organized.	/7
7	I can use multiple types of mnemonic techniques, depending on the situation at hand.	/7
8	I have a list of potential memory palaces written out and add to it regularly.	/7
	TOTAL	/56

In today's world, we are pummeled with an ever-increasing amount of information. The amount of data created, year after year, has been increasing exponentially, yet our brains aren't much different than our ancestors in the dark ages. (Actually, they may have benefited from higher amounts of experiential learning than most schools offer today.)

Nothing can compare to the amount of material you will need to memorize during medical school. And it's not just for a test, but also for your job. Don't worry, we have all been stressed about this at one point or another, but we all got through it (without many of the secrets we're about to share).

Some people are under the false impression that, just because they have heard an individual's name, seen an image, or read a passage once, they will now and forever be the keeper of this knowledge. That's simply not how memory works. Memory is remarkably fluid and plastic, but there are some memory training strategies that can help you to keep memories around for the long haul. Though you can survive medical school without this kind of memory training, learning these techniques will make your life much easier.

If you have the ability, try to master these techniques BEFORE you start medical school. But if you've already started, don't worry! To clarify, these are not magic tricks. They are not tools that only a gifted few can learn to use. They are cognitive strength-training exercises. Some of them may be difficult at first, but this is why we start easy and then work our way up.

Remembering vs. Forgetting

"It is forgetting, not remembering, that is the essence of what makes us human. To make sense of the world, we must filter it."
Joshua Foer

If we are going to talk about how to remember lots of facts, then we ought to know a little bit about what makes us forget. In short, if we do not re-activate and reinforce the neuronal firing patterns that contain the memory, then it will quickly lose strength and eventually be lost. However, it wasn't until Hermann Ebbinghaus formalized the concept of the **Forgetting Curve** that we really started to craft a story about how and why we forget.

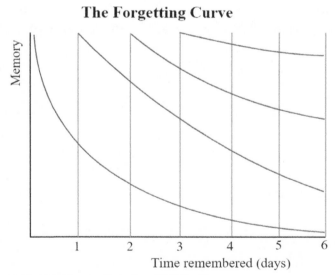

The Forgetting Curve, courtesy of Wikipedia

Ebbinghaus performed many experiments on himself to determine the relationship between time and memory retention. He produced a curve similar to the one seen above. The first curve on the left shows that we can retrieve about half of the information 24 hours later without any practice. By regularly reviewing the information at the point where you expect ~50% loss, you can reinforce the memory and flatten out the Forgetting Curve to promote long-term retention (which is represented by the progression of the other curves on the figure).

It is important to note that the exact dates of when you can expect 50% loss are uncertain (especially past 24 hours), but the principle holds true: Spaced-Repetition fights the Forgetting Curve. Programs like Anki Flashcards, CramFighter and Osmosis use this information to help medical students optimize their study schedules by harnessing the power of Spaced Repetition.

From his data, Ebbinhaus produced a rather complex equation to represent the Forgetting Curve, but more recent work has produced a simpler equation, $R = e^{-t/s}$ [23]. The relationships within this equation are pretty intuitive. Retention of the memory is related to the Strength of the memory and the Time that has passed. Each time you review the material, you essentially reset the clock to $t = zero$ (and reach 100% retention). And to decrease the downward slope of the curve, you need to find a way to Strengthen the memory (e.g., by spaced repetition, active recall, or a mnemonic device).

Now shifting to a discussion of memory itself. We have all heard about short vs. long-term memory. While it's certainly more complicated than a simple binary, for our purposes this schema will work just fine. When actively working through a scenario, the average person can keep track of anywhere from 3 to 9 pieces of cognitive information in their short-term (working) memory. The old rule was 7 +/- 2, which was based on a very famous paper written by George Miller [24].

However, our working memory for specific tasks can significantly improve with training. Anders Ericsson highlights this in his popular book, *Peak*. For months, his test subject was only able to recall 8 random digits in a row. However, with Deliberate Practice, he gradually increased his abilities to >80 digits! Other studies have verified that cognitive training can enhance task-specific working memory [25]. The techniques to boost your memory are being expanded upon each year, which allows memory champions to continue breaking existing records. Nelson Dellis, a 4x US Memory

Champion, explained this while being interviewed on the Medical Mnemonist podcast [26].

Some of the most fascinating research on memory shows how structural changes occur in the brains of people who undergo intensive memory training. A classic experiment showed how prospective London cab drivers who were practicing for their test, referred to as *The Knowledge*, showed growth in areas of the hippocampus related to spatial memory and navigation [27]. Thankfully, less rigorous training programs can produce similar results. In fact, as few as six weeks of training in mnemonic strategies has been linked to stronger functional changes as well, and the effects were seen to last for months [28].

As we have discussed in previous sections, the key to growth in any area is to apply sufficient stress to your faculties, continually pushing yourself beyond your perceived limits. Although we *could* compare memory training to muscle training, the analogy wouldn't be a great one. This is true for many reasons, but for our purposes it's because muscles don't really grow new cells to get bigger and stronger (instead, they increase the size of existing cells). For decades, this was also thought to be true of neurons in the brain, but we now know that humans continually produce new neurons - at least in the hippocampus - to help establish new memories [29,30].

As a final side note for this section, for those of you interested in more extreme cases of memory, consider checking out the story of Clive Wearing, who suffered a severe case of bilateral temporal lobe herpetic encephalopathy [31]. The virus ate away his hippocampi, causing anterograde amnesia. In other words, he could no longer form new memories, so he was given the unfortunate title of, "The Man with the 7-Second Memory."

You could also learn about Kim Peek, whose story was told by the movie *Rain Man*. The memory of Mr. Peek was the closest thing we have ever seen to eidetic "photographic" memory. He memorized thousands of books with nearly perfect recall. When given a memory test, he was able to read 8 pages in 53 seconds and was able to recall the text two hours later with 98.7% accuracy [32].

The (Non)Debate of Multitasking

This section seems to stick out like a sore thumb in the middle of our discussion of memory training and mnemonics, huh? Well, we stuck it here to harken back to some of the pearls we discussed in Part 1 regarding studying and review. Don't forget to apply the tips and tools you've learned thus far to your future readings (including this one). If you're really eager to dive into mnemonics, then skip to the next section. Or you can take a quick tangent with us about multitasking.

Can the average medical student multitask? Short answer: probably not. Multitasking, often by checking your phone while in class or studying, is exceedingly common and impairs your ability to get things done [33]. It is thought to worsen academic performance overall [34]. The issue comes from "task switching," in which going from one task to another takes time and cognitive effort, which slows down task completion. This is sometimes referred to as the "switch cost." Switch costs have been demonstrated to have negative effects on performance even after the stimulus has been taken away [35,36].

So, what does all of this mean for the average learner? **Don't multitask!** When trying to study or get other important work done, put away your phone, silence all alarms, and maybe put on some earmuffs. But on the other end of the spectrum, some in the medical realm still claim that multitasking is a mandatory part of their practice. In fact, emergency medicine physicians undergo formal training for multitasking [37]. If you're going to try this, then you should know ahead of time that multitasking is only useful in a handful of situations.

It's thought that multitasking is really only useful for tasks that do not require significant cognitive load. These kinds of tasks are usually mundane and routine. But, even if you can get two tasks done at once, the performance of one or both will likely suffer [36]. Studying, by definition, is not the kind of task that can be automated because it always requires active engagement with unfamiliar material. Hence, we give a blanket recommendation: don't multitask.

Creating Personal Mnemonics

Now onto another section you have (probably) been looking forward to. Herein we will begin a discussion of mnemonics and memory hacks that make long-term retention easier. In medicine, we mostly use acronyms and initialism, such as CSF for cerebrospinal fluid. Another good example would be MRSA (methicillin-resistant staphylococcus aureus). Though some people say M-R-S-A, others pronounce it as a word: "Mrsa."

Acronyms and initialism are relatively easy to use as memory tools on the fly (e.g., PVT TIM HALL to remember the essential amino acids: phenylalanine, valine, tryptophan, threonine, isoleucine, methionine, histidine, arginine, lysine, leucine). The problem is, they are relatively weak memory devices. You will never hear a memory champion bragging about the cool acronyms they came up with. They are rarely visual, nor are they personalized. So, even though they can be passed down from one student to the next, you have very little *personal* attachment to them.

Their use MAY get you through your next biochem exam, but the majority of these mnemonics are forgotten a few weeks later. We would *guesstimate* that the average student could hold on to 5% of these types of mnemonics over the long haul. Unfortunately, this probably won't cut it for the boards, and it certainly won't help for the rest of your career.

You could spend time putting them on flashcards and using spaced repetition to remember them better. But, that's so passé! So, we would argue that these mnemonic devices can be useful in a pinch for low-yield details that you expect to see on an in-class exam, but for higher-yield information you should use a stronger technique instead. While these stronger techniques are probably less familiar, we would argue that they produce better results (and they are more fun).

The key to advanced memory techniques is the visual marker. Anyone that has seen a Sketchy Medical video or Picmonic scene is aware of the power of imagery (and storytelling) when memorizing seemingly disjointed facts. These visual cues will "mark" a certain topic, word, number, or process with an easily associated visual mnemonic.

But, what if, instead of paying a third-party company, you could learn how to do this yourself? Creating visual markers and memory palaces are skills that have been practiced since antiquity. Think about those stories you may have heard of monks memorizing vast stretches of holy texts. There was really nothing special about their brains. It's not *that* hard to do, but it will take some effort/training upfront.

Unfortunately, the exact methods used by these ancient mnemonists weren't clearly recorded, so it's taken some trial and error to develop effective systems. Thankfully, others have put in the hard work for you. The 8-time World Memory Champion, Dominic O'Brien, has put together a number of books, games, and other learning materials for the fledgling mnemonist. The Dominic System is usually credited as the precursor to the even more powerful PAO System, which will be discussed soon.

In one of his earlier works, *Quantum Memory Power*, O'Brien states there are three parts to a powerful memory: **Association**, **Location**, and **Imagination**. This provides the framework from which we will create our future mnemonics.

Supplementing this mental framework, Dr. Aaron Nelson, author of *Harvard Medical School Guide to Achieving Optimal Memory,* identifies the four main "ingredients" for a sticky mnemonic: 1) unique experiences, 2) use the five senses, 3) make it meaningful, and 4) add emotion. As we can see from this list, it is difficult for pre-made mnemonics to be as meaningful to us as *de novo* visual marker mnemonics. However, if you are going to use pre-made images, try to add in these ingredients where possible to make the memory stronger and fight the ever-lurking Forgetting Curve.

If you watch the Memory Championships, you can see for yourself just how effective they are. Honestly, you don't actually *want* to watch this kind of competition because it's supremely boring from an outsider's perspective; all the excitement is taking place in the minds of the competitors. Rather, try it out for yourself by simply looking up a few memory demonstration videos.

You may be thinking, "But I have three quizzes, two assignments, and a presentation coming up. I don't have time to train like this." We hear you. And this may seem like a daunting task, but we regret that we didn't find out about it sooner. If you're going to give it a shot, there's no time like the present. Again, learning to produce your own mnemonics is important for two key reasons: 1) personalized imagery increases the strength/duration of the memory, and 2) it is a lifelong skill that can be used in nearly any context.

Let's tackle these points one at a time. To make an image personalized, the scene only needs to make sense to *you*. Just think about it. If someone else were to describe the scene of a patient encounter, this will only produce a superficial memory on your end. But your own encounters are much more vivid and long-lasting.

Bolstering this point, we have interviewed a bunch of memory champions on the Medical Mnemonist podcast, and all of them agree: *for the best results, you have to create your own personalized images.* If you study someone else's mnemonics, you do not have the connection to the material.

Yes, learning to produce your own scenes will take time. Like learning a new language, the first few words and sentences are the most difficult. But after that, you start to get a hold of the syntax and grammar, to expand your vocabulary, and to gain confidence in your new skills. If you cannot find any time to practice during the academic year, then holiday breaks could be a good time to start. If you want to listen to an example of Chase and Greg actively creating a memory palace together, check out their joint episode on the Medical Mnemonist podcast.

The second reason we advocate for personalized mnemonics is that developing this skill will be useful far beyond medical school. It can be adapted to EVERY part of your life. For example, it can help you remember the names of other students, physicians, nurses, and staff during your rotations and residency. It can be applied to your specialty boards and re-certification exams. These techniques can even be used to assist in remembering important dates, grocery lists, account numbers, etc.

To begin this practice, there are multiple exercises you can choose to start with, and they will be explored in greater detail soon. Initially, there are different tools for names, numbers, language, etc. But, **the more you practice, the easier it is to mix and match techniques for greater impact**. You'll probably gravitate towards one technique to start with, then branch out and experiment from there.

One last comment before we begin: have fun with it! If you approach these like a chore, they will become one. If you approach this like a quest or game, it will be much more enjoyable. Eliminating the stress associated with learning/practice can help to open up your creativity and allow for stronger associations to be made.

Creativity, Visual Mnemonics, and other Memory Tools

How do most of us try to memorize information? Some people like to use flash cards or repetitive drilling. Others like to read and re-read their study notes. Still others like to use more creative techniques like drawing mind maps. All of these approaches have their place. But most of them, especially re-reading study notes, tend not to produce robust long-term memories. At best, they get us through the next exam. In our experience, the best tool for students memorizing information for the long term is the **visual mnemonic**.

Visual mnemonics harness our innate ability to store visual information for the long term. Think about it: you can probably remember many of the famous scenes from your favorite movies or TV shows. Or you can easily picture the living room from your childhood home. These memories are remarkably long-lived and vivid. In contrast, it is extremely difficult for most of us to memorize a few lines on a page or note card. While text on a page is a highly efficient way to *externally* store data for the long term, we know that our memories just don't connect to it very well.

One exception to this rule is the use of rhyme, rhythm, or poetic cadence to link together a string of words. For example, you can easily remember the words to your favorite songs, right? Hence, with accelerated learning techniques and mnemonics, all we are trying to do is to take advantage of inborn human strengths. Why go against our nature when trying to memorize important information?

Not everyone has a knack for creating memorable rhymes or lyrics, but just about every can visualize a scene in their head. Hence, we will focus on creating visual mnemonics. If you've ever done this before, you know that creating mnemonics can be a fun way to get your creative juices flowing. Even if years of rigid classroom instruction have dulled your creative edge, you have not lost everything! From a research perspective, there are plenty of theoretical frameworks that describe the creative process. For our purposes, we will consider the work by Graham Wallace. In his classic piece, *The Art of Thought*, Wallace proposes a 4-stage model for creativity: Preparation, Incubation, Illumination, and Verification [38].

In Preparation, we define the problem or desired outcome. In Incubation we allow our mind to ruminate over the issue. In Illumination, we consolidate our ideas and solutions. In Verification, we test our ideas to see if they work.

This simple model can be used to describe the creation of just about anything, including visual mnemonics. What is a visual mnemonic? A visual mnemonic is a mental scene that has various *visual markers* in it, which stand in for pieces of data that you want to memorize. By clustering the data together into a scene, you allow for easier long-term association of the data by a phenomenon known as mental chunking. The Wikipedia entry for mental chunking actually describes the phenomenon quite well [39]:

"Chunking is a process by which individual pieces of an information set are broken down and then grouped together in a meaningful whole... These chunks are able to be retrieved more easily due to their coherent familiarity... The items are more easily remembered as a group than as the individual items themselves."

Visual mnemonics take advantage of our innate abilities to both chunk information and retain images in long-term memory. If the idea of a visual mnemonic sounds familiar, you may have heard of it under a different name like a Memory Palace (recently popularized by the modern British TV drama, *Sherlock*). Visual mnemonics are essentially the same thing as memory palaces.

In the small world of medical education, there are excellent products already on the market, like Sketchy Medical or Picmonic, that have created visual mnemonics that help medical students to study memorization-heavy subjects like microbiology and pharmacology. But you don't necessarily need to *pay* for these resources. Instead, you have the ability to make your own visual mnemonics *de novo*. It just takes time, effort, and a little bit of creativity to learn this skill.

When you're in the middle of medical school and drinking from the *information firehose*, it may feel overwhelming commit yourself to learning a new skill like this, so we would recommend trying this out before you begin your pre-clinical studies (if possible). That being said, if you're motivated, you can master this skill at any point in your career.

How can we learn to create our own visual mnemonics? We will begin with a silly example. Let's say that we wanted to remember how Watson and Crick discovered the genome in 1953. Chase actually used this mnemonic in a previous blog post called *Memory Palaces for Medical Students* [40].

> Imagine Lt. Watson from Sherlock Holmes with a little cricket sitting on his shoulder. Suddenly, a bat flies into the scene and snatches up the cricket in its claws, leaving behind a patch of blood on Watson's jacket.

So, how does this all come together? We first decided on the raw data: Watson & Crick, 1953, genome. Then we let the concept incubate for some time to come up with creative visual markers that could be brought together into a single, personally memorable scene. Illumination suggested that the scene called for a gruesome element - the predatory bat swooping in to eat the cricket - which helps to make the mnemonic more emotionally salient.

The tricky part is creating a hook for 1953. Perhaps you could imagine Watson inspecting Clue Number 53 or he could be knocking on the door of 1953 Baker Street. Be as original or unoriginal as you want. You don't need to have a clear system worked out for every contingency before you begin. **Just get started!** Later on, you will be able to add to your "visual dictionary" and use your pre-made visual markers to add more consistency (and flair) to your scenes.

The Verification step would come if, at a later time, the scene was recalled and the information was retrieved (or not). Of course, spaced-retrieval practice and other factors play a part. But this exercise demonstrates the creation of a simple visual mnemonic.

Start with something that's low pressure. For example, you could pick a few facts from a random book or article that you'd like to commit to memory. Once you start to get the hang of it, you can actually have a lot of fun doing this (in a nerdy way). Once you are motivated to keep using the technique, you can be comforted by the fact that intrinsic motivation actually boosts your creativity [41], which forms a positive-feedback cycle for learning. This correlates with a concept described in the book *Flow*: enjoyment of the activity, not the reward, gives the best results.

One last thing to help invigorate your creative juices is the **SCAMPER** tool. This stands for: Substitute, Combine, Adapt, Modify, Put to another use, Eliminate, and Reverse. This brainstorming tool can be used to elicit new ideas when creating visual markers, modifying existing ones, or for any other creative purpose. Even a simple change to the shape, size, color or direction can help to make a bland marker more memorable.

Hopefully, this primer section has piqued your interest. Now let's dig a little bit deeper into some of the mnemonic devices that you can develop as a part of your memory toolbox.

Basics of Visual Markers

Visual markers are a type of mental visual aid that we can place into our visual mnemonics, like our scene with Lt. Watson and his Cricket. When starting your practice with visual markers, one good heuristic to follow is that **the first image is the best**. If you want to convert a fact into a visual marker, the first thing that comes to mind is likely your strongest visual association to that topic. It's already there. Just use it.

For example, think about the word, "microbiology." What comes to mind?... You may picture a microscope, a researcher in a lab coat, a bacterial culture growing, or maybe a cartoon depiction of a bacterium. These are great places to start. Or maybe your first impression was more *vivid*: an infected/necrotic diabetic foot wound; a video clip of a white blood cell chasing a bacterium around a petri dish; or even a funny meme that you saw about bacteria. (It's okay. This is a safe space.)

Whatever the visual, there is a reason that image came to mind. If *nothing* comes to mind or the association is too weak - which is more common with new subjects and difficult words - there are a bunch of different angles you can take.

Play on Words: If the word rhymes or sounds similar to another (more memorable) word, then use this connection. You can also try to associate numbers with objects. For example, the number 1 kind of looks like a pencil. So, in your visual mnemonic, you could use a pencil to represent the number one. In the section on the Peg System (below), you will find a table full of visual markers for numbers.

Etymology: Sometimes, finding the root and history of a word can provide inspiration for a visual marker. Try typing the difficult word into the Online Etymology Dictionary. You might be surprised by what you find. For instance, did you know the word avocado can be traced back to the word testicle? [42] You could also check out a crowdsourced databank of mnemonics like MnemonicDictionary.com.

Sound it Out: For particularly long or complex words, try breaking them down syllable by syllable. We can use Dr. Csikszentmihalyi's name - the author of *Flow* - for our example. "Csik-szent-mi-halyi" kind of sounds like "chat set me high" when spoken rapidly. You could then convert the name into a scene, such as a *chatting* construction worker who is *setting* concrete. He's chatting with *me*, and I'm sitting *high* up in the building rafters.

Make it Absurd: If your visual aid is weak or rather *plain vanilla*, you can spice things up by manipulating some of the details. For example, rather than picturing a simple apple or a fidget spinner, picture a tie-dye apple with a funky worm coming out, or imagine a fidget spinner that spins so fast it begins to take off into space! These exaggerations make a deeper impact precisely because they are out of the ordinary. The brain will usually purge mundane details from our daily lives - like what you had for breakfast 8 days ago - so don't be afraid to make it absurd. This kind of divergent thinking tends to decrease as we age [43]. Keep yourself fresh by expanding your mental horizons.

*If you find this list of mnemonic hacks to be insufficient, try Googling for more ideas or try to create your own. You do you. And feel free to share your experiences, or seek feedback, on the Medical Mnemonist Mastermind Facebook group. As we've pointed out multiple times now, just get started. Experimentation is the name of the game.

Memorizing Numbers

Now, how can we use mnemonics to remember numbers, like epidemiology stats or reference values for labs? Probably the easiest method we know of is the **Peg System**. This system was originally used to memorize strings of random numbers, but you can adapt it to suit your needs as a medical student.

Below is a sample Peg System. Each digit is associated with a visual marker that *sounds* like, *looks* like, or *seems* like that digit. Feel free to use this table or to make your own. By associating specific visual markers to numbers, the average person can boost themselves from remembering 7 digits in a row (typical phone number) to 20+ numbers in a row. For optimal results, you ought to link the visual markers together into a story that makes sense.

See chart on the following page

Peg System	Rhyme- "sounds like"	Shape- "looks like"	Associate- "seems like"
1	Gun	Pen/Pencil	Snowboard (Vs Skis)
2	Shoe	Swan Neck	Ears/Eyes/Etc.
3	Key, Tree	Bat Flying	Tricycle
4	Door	Chair	Car Tires
5	Hive	Hanger/Hook	Hand/Glove (5 Fingers)
6	Sticks, Licks	Yo-yo on String	Sextuplets
7	Evan, Even	Stickle/Hockey Stick	Seven Society (Secret Organization)
8	Skates	Race Track, glasses	Stop Sign (Octagon)
9	Supine	Blossoming Flower	Cat (9 Lives)
10	Big Ben	Ring(o)	Bowling Pins, 10-sided Dice

For our example of Lt. Watson and his unfortunate cricket, you might remember the year 1953 by having Watson pull his gun (one) and diving onto his back (supine) to take aim with a steady hand (five) at the predatory flying bat (three) that attacked his cricket.

Creating and memorizing a table such as this can be very helpful for remembering practical things like your new phone number, as well as medical knowledge like the frequency of certain diseases.

Pro tip: having multiple objects makes it easier to remember longer strings. Otherwise, a sequence like 11341 would have pencils flying everywhere! You can always search online for more creative ideas on how to fill in your visual marker table. Whatever system you choose, make sure to write it down in a journal for safekeeping.

If you don't like the Peg System, there is another system known as the Major Method or Major System. This converts numbers into sounds, which you then associate with words. The sounds were chosen by its creator, Aimé Paris, and must simply be memorized for this method to work. Here are the sounds that are associated with the digits 0-10:

Major System / Major Method										
0	1	2	3	4	5	6	7	8	9	10
c, s, z	d, t, th	n	m	r	l	ch, j, sh, or soft g	k, q, hard c, or hard g	f, v, ph	p, b	X

This method is much less intuitive than the Peg System, but it is highly praised by some memory champions for its utility. Maybe they're the best Scrabble players of the bunch? Anyway, you may notice that there are no vowels in this chart. This gives you the ability to add in vowels wherever you wish to make a word out of the associated sounds. Once you have the table memorized, you can turn 09285807437013102712 into spnfl-f-sgr-mks-t-mtcn-g-dn, which is loosely translated into, "A spoonful of sugar makes the medicine go down."

You may decide that committing one of these systems to memory isn't worth the hassle during medical school, but knowing that **you have options available** is usually reassuring. There are plenty of other ways to harness your creativity when studying.

If you do decide to commit a number system to memory, practice by using an online random number generator to make a string of digits. Then create a story with all of your visual markers in it. Then look away from the number string and try to recite the story (and try to recite the numbers in the string). If you can do this consistently, then you're a pro and you'll have no trouble filling your brain with fun stats. To keep your visual marker table fresh, try recreating it from memory every couple of weeks. Remember: with memories, if you don't use 'em, you lose 'em!

Memorizing Names and Faces

Many people have trouble putting a name to a face. As Dale Carnegie says in his classic book, *How to Win Friends and Influence People*, "A person's name is to that person, the sweetest, most important sound in any language." Forgetting a person's name can be terribly embarrassing, especially in the professional world. When trying to remember a new acquaintance's name in the moment, you can reinforce your memory by intentionally using their name multiple times in the conversation (just don't be awkward about it). Beyond that, you can use some of the following strategies:

Name to a Place: If you have more difficulty with their name than their face, you may use this basic technique. Let's bring back our Dr. Csikszentmihalyi mnemonic from before. We used the Sound-it-Out method to remember how to pronounce his name (roughly coming out to *chat-set-me-high*) which we converted to a scene with a chatty construction worker who was setting concrete and talking to me as I sit high above him. But what if we wanted to remember his face instead? Perhaps he is in the visual of the construction yard or he even becomes the chatty construction worker setting the concrete. This method has no rules, so get creative with your associations. Again, whatever association your mind comes up with *first* is likely going to be a solid first step.

Face to a Place: With this strategy, you want to match the person to a location. Do you get the feeling that they look like a librarian, mechanic, boxer, lawyer, receptionist, etc.? Use this unconscious association to your advantage! Insert his/her face into a scene where you would find such a person. You can then add in a visual marker that will be associated with their name. For instance, if your charge nurse, Georgia, looks like a librarian, then try picture her at your local library. Place a map on the wall behind her with the state of Georgia circled. Or maybe she's eating a Georgia peach in the library? For another example, if you think Jack from HR looks like a mechanic, then you could visualize him in an auto mechanic's shop *jacking* up a car.

Associated Person: You might find it easiest to associate the new individual to someone you already are familiar with that holds the same name. Associating the new Rob at work to your Uncle Rob may give a host of potential connections to explore. For example, work Rob and Uncle Rob may share a hobby like fishing, so you could imagine them fishing together. Alternatively, you might imagine them *robbing* a bank together. Don't worry, nobody will know about these visual markers but you.

Prominent Feature: To really drill down on the face of your new acquaintance, try focusing on a prominent feature, such as their nose, eyes, eyebrows, ears, moles, blemishes, etc. Then try to associate that feature with their name in some fashion. If your supervisor, Reese, has particularly large ears, try to visual her wearing Reese's candy bars as earrings. We've only provided a few examples above, but as you can imagine, the possibilities are plentiful.

Beyond social acquaintances, the tactics above can also be used to remember *eponymously named diseases* (i.e., diseases which are named after the discoverer or a famous case). Medicine is slowly but steadily moving away from eponymous disease names, like Lou Gehrig's, towards more descriptive names like Amyotrophic Lateral Sclerosis.

There's also a wealth of tutorial videos online for more examples. You may wish to start your practice by searching out images and names of random people online, or even going out in public to associate a stranger's face to a new location. (Just don't be creepy about it!) For *extreme* memory training, some even recommend taking a course on face drawing so that you can be more aware of the subtle differences that make a face unique.

Regardless of whether you use the specific techniques above, it will be important for you to **keep a record of your mnemonics** and to build time into your day to recall previous mnemonics (and check your recall against your records). Adding a basic sketch of the mnemonic into your notes can be a great addition to your study materials. A written description is fine if drawing out the mnemonic proves too cumbersome.

Memory Palaces

The previous sections previewed some of the basic techniques for creating visual markers. However, learning how to use these in a study session and for long-term memorization can be challenging. Ultimately, it just takes time to experiment and find what works best.

One of the first strategies you may wish to use is the memory palace. What is a memory palace? Similar to a visual mnemonic, it's a mental space where you place visual markers to represent information that you want to memorize. Memory palaces take advantage of our natural ability to remember visual scenes in great detail. Remember that your technique will be constantly evolving so there is no *right* or *wrong* way of using a memory palace.

The setting for your memory palaces should be places that you are very familiar with. For example, you could use your past or current home, homes of friends and family members, school buildings, restaurants, offices, stores, parks, streets, whatever. You could even search homes on Zillow and create a memory palace based on the images from the seller. The key is to use locations that you can reliably picture in great detail. For a live example of how to create a memory palace (for cephalosporin antibiotics), check out this podcast episode on the Medical Mnemonist featuring Chase and Greg [44].

Now, let's build a memory palace together. To keep things easy, select your bedroom for the location. Close your eyes and look around the room in your *mind's eye*. Note the different pieces of furniture, fixtures, pictures, closet space, and anything else that could be used as a location to drop a visual marker. Sketch out or list the stations (or loci) you will use. We recommend 3-6 loci per palace (as a ballpark figure). If you need more markers for the topic, consider using multiple rooms. Alternatively, you can have multiple markers sharing one locus in the room.

Now it's time to come up with visual markers to represent the information you need to memorize. As we mentioned in a previous section, the easiest way to start is to think of wordplay and rhymes. If it's a long word or technical term, you may wish to break it into pieces by syllables. Then use these syllables to create visual markers.

After you have created your visual markers, it's time to arrange them around the room at the various loci. For example, there may be a hierarchy of importance among the markers at locus 1 vs. locus 2 vs. locus 3, etc. If there's no clear hierarchy, use whatever sequence comes to your mind first. A common approach is to move about the room in a clockwise fashion to each locus, but it all depends on how your brain wants to encode the information.

> *Note from Greg: Sketch out each station of the memory palace as you create them. Add notes and further description where needed. Try to recall each palace from start to finish on a semi-regular basis (and check yourself against your records). Doing so will help to fight the Forgetting Curve!*

Congratulations! You have just gone through the steps to make a memory palace. Your first few palaces will be mentally taxing to construct. However, here's one piece of good news: any visual markers you make can easily be reused in future memory palaces. For example, if you use the image of a *sink full of peas* to represent the symptom of *syncope*, then you could easily reuse that visual marker for future memory palaces. You might have the sink of peas in a palace for the side effects of beta-blockers, as well as a palace for the differential diagnosis of seizures. Over time, you'll develop a **Visual Marker Dictionary**. As this dictionary grows, it becomes easier to produce new palaces.

Just remember, memory champions are called "mental athletes" for a reason. These skills take time and practice to develop (ideally Deliberate Practice). Every learner will come to points where they feel stuck. When you hit a roadblock, don't hesitate to seek help from a study buddy or mentor. You could also solicit feedback and advice from the Medical Mnemonist Mastermind Facebook group. Or you could check out some of the episodes of the Medical Mnemonist Podcast, which invites memory athletes and medical educators alike to share their pearls of wisdom.

For example, Anthony Metivier [45] explains how he uses his CREAT and CURE methods to organize and elaborate within his palaces. He also has a free course that all newcomers can start with. Similarly, Ryan Orwig elaborated on his experiences teaching medical students how to use accelerated learning techniques, such as his Minimally Effective Linking strategy [46].

As you develop your skills, try applying them to more complicated materials. Medical podcasts, research journals, and even your class lectures can be converted into dynamic visual creations on the fly. Have a great idea, but you're unable to write it down? Create a quick visual marker and place it in a temporary palace for later recall. There's virtually no limitation to when or where these skills may come in handy.

Note from Chase: I have a lot of thoughts while driving, meditating, or am otherwise unable to write things down. Using visual markers, I can place images and scenes in a location in my home for later recall. For example, when meditating I may place them on the furniture in front of me. That way, when I open my eyes at the end of the meditation the associated furniture will prompt the image.

Practical Tips from the Experts

Memory champions caution that novice memory palace builders tend to make similar mistakes. Alex Mullen and Cathy Chen, both of whom are memory athletes (and physicians), observed that one of the most common mistakes is trying to squeeze too many visual markers into a single memory palace [47]. This is more likely to happen when you are new to the material, or if you have not developed your mnemonic skills.

Let's use this excerpt from the Wikipedia page on *Staphylococcus aureus* to illustrate the point [48]:

> Staphylococcus aureus is a Gram-positive, round-shaped bacterium that is a member of the Firmicutes, and it is a usual member of the microbiota of the body, frequently found in the upper respiratory tract and on the skin. It is often positive for catalase and nitrate reduction and is a facultative anaerobe that can grow without the need for oxygen. Although S. aureus usually acts as a commensal of the human microbiota it can also become an opportunistic pathogen, being a common cause of skin infections including abscesses, respiratory infections such as sinusitis, and food poisoning.
>
> S. aureus can cause a range of illnesses, from minor skin infections, such as pimples, impetigo, boils, cellulitis, folliculitis, carbuncles, scalded skin syndrome, and abscesses, to life-threatening diseases such as pneumonia, meningitis, osteomyelitis, endocarditis, toxic shock syndrome, bacteremia, and sepsis.

There is A LOT of information packed into this short block of text and all of it is board-testable. We could make a marker for the microbe itself, one for its gram-positive nature, one for the shape, and so on. However, if we were to make a visual marker for each key point, our palace would be quickly overrun! Now imagine applying that to the thousands of pages for each textbook of your curriculum. This issue can be avoided with a little bit of preparation.

There is no need to make a visual marker for every single fact. Your innate ability to organize and mentally chunk the material can take you very far [39]. Instead, you should only plan to make markers and memory palaces for material that is particularly difficult for *you* to remember. Your professors should already help to categorize/organize the material in their lecture slides and readings, which makes your job much easier. If you want to re-categorize later, it shouldn't be too hard. Just don't go trying to fix something that isn't broken.

If it is a completely new area of study, it may be best to take notes first and translate them into your memory palace later. Alternatively, you could plan to preview the next day's lectures, book chapter, etc. ahead of time. The purpose is not to memorize the content yet, but to get a feel for the key terms, the quantity, and the overall structure. For example, if the text has 12 subsections, you should plan on having at least this many loci spread across your memory palaces. If each subsection is very dense, you may need to plan for more than one palace per subsection.

For a topic like Staph infections of the skin, you could plan to set up a memory palace with loci for signs/symptoms (red, warm, swollen, tender), features of MSSA vs. MRSA (antibiotic resistance), diagnostic tests (nasal PCR or skin culture), and treatments (antibiotics like mupirocin, oxacillin, cefazolin, cefalexin, Bactrim, clindamycin, doxycycline, etc.). Notice how each locus would need to store multiple visual markers.

If time allows, consider investigating some of the companies that produce visual mnemonic software. Currently, Picmonic offers a self-directed Picmonic Generator [49]. Sketchy Medical and Physeo also have great products to offer. In general, we would recommend that you try to create your own visual markers and memory palaces because they tend to be more distinct/memorable. But you can certainly draw a lot of inspiration from existing products on the market.

As you get better at creating memory palaces, you might even be able to make them on the fly *during* lecture. This will be easier if you have previewed the material and are well-prepared for the class. As a part of your preparation, you could try to sketch out a basic outline of the palace ahead of time, then fine-tune it based on the material your professor emphasizes.

Finally, remember to have fun. Mnemonics are easier to make when the mind is free and loose. Excess stress can kill creativity [50], so don't feel like you need to force yourself to make a memory palace for every subject. If it's producing anxiety, then take a break and try an alternate approach. A memory palace is simply another tool in your arsenal; *you decide* when and how to use it.

Advanced Memory Training Techniques

To be as complete as possible, we wanted to add a brief section on more advanced techniques for memory training. Though many of the details are beyond the scope of this book, being aware of the ever-evolving techniques used by memory athletes may assist in your scholarly endeavors.

The **Dominic System** [51] from creator and 8-time memory champion, Dominic O'Brien, is a classic among memory athlete circles. It was originally developed to help users rapidly memorize a sequence of playing cards or random digits. Basically, the user would create a unique marker for each of the 52 cards in a deck or for each of the first 100 whole numbers.

For example, the eighth letter of the alphabet is H, so he associated the number 88 with the visual marker of Hulk Hogan (HH for 88). Now, let's say you wanted to memorize a string of digits, like 884432. You could picture Hulk Hogan putting Daffy Duck (DD for 44) into a chokehold; Daffy then counters by swinging a Close Band radio at Hogan's head (CB for 32) in order to get free.

As you can imagine, the Dominic System can be remarkably flexible and useful in a variety of situations. O'Brien attributes much of his success to using it. However, his system has limitations. Later practitioners have upgraded to the **Person-Action-Object (PAO) System** [52].

The more contemporary/advanced 3-digit PAO System allows for even greater flexibility, but it requires more effort up front. Memory athletes will memorize a three-column chart from 000-999 where the first digit is a Person, the second digit is an Action, and the third digit is an Object being acted upon. (You can also change the order from PAO to POA to OPA, etc.)

Will you ever need to memorize absurdly long strings of numbers in your studies or future occupation? No. And dedicating enough time to memorize your own PAO chart probably won't be worth it for medical school. But, it is clear that the human mind is capable of amazing feats if we keep it organized and dedicated. There's nothing intrinsically unique about the brains of these memory athletes; it's all about the training. Perhaps you can utilize a strategy like this to memorize drugs, microbes, biochemical pathways, etc?

If you're ever "stuck" and unable to create a sticky mnemonic, know there are plenty of options and resources available. For example, color coding and adding emotion to visual markers are great ways to make subtle distinctions between facts. Including all of your natural senses (sight, sound, taste, touch, smell) can add more vividness to the mnemonic. Some researchers even suggest that, with practice, we can develop synesthesia-like skills [53]. We might even be able to connect our visual markers from a wide range of fields to produce new insights for research or personal connection, which is what the Hyperlinking Technique strives to do [54].

The only limitation is your own creativity and the creativity of those you surround yourself with. Thankfully (or not), with the internet, we can expand our circle to anyone who is willing to post online. You can get plenty of inspiration from a community of like-minded individuals. For example, the Medical Mnemonist Facebook group would be a great place to start.

Mind Mapping

Mind Maps are a creation of memory guru, Tony Buzan. They are a great way to organize your thoughts, schedules, and study materials in a visually creative manner (see example below). By creating a visually-organized mind map, you can more easily identify links and associations between disparate topics [55]. They take a form similar to that of a concept map, with the main topic in the center of the page. Sub-topics sprout from the main topic using colorful pathways and graphics. These sub-topics can have branches of their own, which can connect and interact with other branches in the mind map.

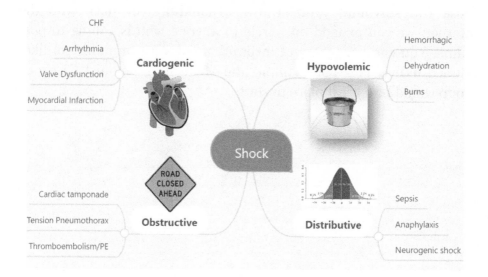

The key difference between Mind Maps and other graphic organizers is the intentional addition of visual markers like the ones used in memory palaces. Strategically placing these visual markers makes it easier for the learner to recreate the mind map from memory.

Effective use of Mind Maps has been shown to improve factual recall [56] and is associated with higher levels of creativity [57]. However, results are mixed and few studies have been conducted comparing well-trained mind map users when compared to other study strategies. One study performed among medical students showed that, for novices, mind maps didn't seem to make much difference, but it certainly didn't hurt [58]. So, mind maps could be a useful alternative for your studies if regular note-taking just isn't cutting it.

We suggest you use whatever note-taking strategy you feel comfortable with. But if you have the time and the inclination, try making a mind map; it can be pretty fun! Consider placing these drawings around your room for quick reminders, or take a photo which can be put into a flashcard deck for later review.

We would generally advise *against* using commercial software when making your own mind maps. While they can produce very neat images, they are slow and clunky to use. Slow and clunky are not compatible with the lifestyle of a medical student. Also, by drawing out your own maps by hand, you can usually be more creative with structure/formatting. Mind maps are a great supplement to your existing study methods. For a quick tutorial, check out this video. And for a more professional example, check out this one.

Closing Thoughts - Part 3

No matter what, you will have finite memory and recall. Much of our cognitive limitations are probably related to genetic differences, disease/damage, and other factors out of our control. Worrying about what you can't remember is much less important than praising yourself for the things you can. If you have trouble staying mindful of your small successes with each day, try getting into the habit of keeping a gratitude journal. Excessive anxiety about your own "short-comings" will only decrease your performance on the boards and wards. Just do your best; beyond that, nobody can reasonably ask for more from you.

The tools we've provided in this section can give your studies a boost. Not all of them will work for each person, but there is great value in testing them out to see which techniques will jive with your learning style. None of them will be a silver bullet, but every little bit can help. Just like anything you practice, you can only expect to reap what you sow. **Go get started!** And if you're already in the midst of practicing some of these techniques, think back to our discussion of Deliberate Practice to find ways to maximize your results.

In Part 4, the last section of this book, we will reinforce the point that regular self-assessment is crucial for your future growth. Within this context, we will quickly review many of the high-yield tips and tricks that we have shared thus far. This review will be supported by concrete examples that can take your understanding beyond abstractions. Also, because we have harped on journaling quite a bit, we will give you a brief explanation of why we feel it's so valuable. We hope that you've enjoyed reading this text, that you have found value within its pages, and that we will play a small part in shaping your fantastic future career.

References - Part 3

References can also be found at https://freemeded.org/book-references/

1. Maguire EA et al. (2003) Routes to remembering: the brains behind superior memory. URL: https://www.nature.com/articles/nn988

2. Dresler M et al. (2017) Mnemonic training reshapes brain networks to support superior memory. URL: https://www.cell.com/neuron/fulltext/S0896-6273(17)30087-9?_returnURL=https%3A%2F%2Flinkinghub.elsevier.com%2Fretrieve%2Fpii%2FS0896627317300879%3Fshowall%3Dtrue

3. Some well known speed readers. URL: http://www.readfaster.com/articles/well-known-speed-readers.asp

4. Key to Study website. URL: http://www.keytostudy.com/examplary-training-schedule/

5. Marczyk J. (2017) The adaptive significance of priming. URL: https://www.psychologytoday.com/us/blog/pop-psych/201701/the-adaptive-significance-priming

6. Dingler T et al. (2015) Utilizing the effects of priming to facilitate text comprehension. URL: https://www.researchgate.net/publication/300725105_Utilizing_the_Effects_of_Priming_to_Facilitate_Text_Comprehension

7. Vanderline W. (2018) Speed reading: Fact or fiction? URL: https://www.csicop.org/index.php/si/show/speed_reading_fact_or_fiction

8. Waterloo Student Success Office. Speed Reading Handout. URL: https://uwaterloo.ca/student-success/sites/ca.student-success/files/uploads/files/TipSheet_SpeedReading.pdf

9. Payne BR et al. (2017) Out of the corner of my eye: Foveal semantic load modulates parafoveal processing in reading. URL: https://www.ncbi.nlm.nih.gov/pmc/articles/PMC5083148/

10. Schotter ER et al. (2012) Parafoveal processing in reading. URL: https://link.springer.com/article/10.3758/s13414-011-0219-2

11. Key to Study, Visual Angle Training page. URL: http://www.keytostudy.com/visual-angle-training/

12. Howard Berg Interview. URL: https://medicalmnemonist.podbean.com/e/speed-learning-with-guinness-world-speed-reading-record-holder-howard-berg/

13. Key to Study, Subvocalization page. URL: http://www.keytostudy.com/subvocalization-suppression-training/

14. Ibbotson M & Krekelberg B. (2011) Visual perception and saccadic eye movements. URL: https://www.ncbi.nlm.nih.gov/pmc/articles/PMC3175312/

15. University of Cambridge, MRC Cognition and Brain Sciences Unit website. URL: https://www.mrc-cbu.cam.ac.uk/people/matt.davis/cmabridge/

16. Starrfelt R et al. (2013) Don't words come easy? A psychophysical exploration of word superiority. URL: https://www.ncbi.nlm.nih.gov/pmc/articles/PMC3761163/

17. Morrison AB et al. (2014) Primacy and recency effects as indices of the focus of attention. URL: https://www.ncbi.nlm.nih.gov/pmc/articles/PMC3900765/

18. Sand K et al. (2016) The word superiority effect in central and peripheral vision. URL: https://www.tandfonline.com/doi/abs/10.1080/13506285.2016.1259192

19. Moshtael H et al. (2016) Saccadic scrolling: Speed reading strategy based on natural eye movements. URL: https://ieeexplore.ieee.org/abstract/document/7783909

20. Kumari V et al. (2017) The mindful eye: Smooth pursuit and saccadic eye movements in meditators and non-meditators. URL: https://www.sciencedirect.com/science/article/pii/S1053810016302100

21. Key to Study, Speed Reading. URL: http://www.keytostudy.com/ten-common-speedreading-mistakes/

22. Abdullah M. (2018) Reading speed and comprehension enhancement in hybrid learning delivery mode. URL: http://journals.aiac.org.au/index.php/alls/article/view/4511/3484

23. Murre JM & Dros J. (2015) Replication and analysis of Ebbinghaus' Forgetting Curve. URL: https://www.ncbi.nlm.nih.gov/pmc/articles/PMC4492928/

24. Miller GA (1955) The magical number seven, plus or minus two: Some limits on our capacity for processing information. URL: http://www2.psych.utoronto.ca/users/peterson/psy430s2001/Miller%20GA%20Magical%20Seven%20Psych%20Review%201955.pdf

25. Schmiedek F et al. (2010) Hundreds of days of cognitive training enhance broad cognitive abilities in adulthood: Findings from the COGITO study. URL: https://www.ncbi.nlm.nih.gov/pmc/articles/PMC2914582/

26. Nelson Dellis Interview. URL: https://medicalmnemonist.podbean.com/e/visual-marker-creation-journey-method-w-nelson-dellis-climb4memory-4x-us-memory-champion-and-author/

27. Woollett K & Maguire EA. (2011) Acquiring "the Knowledge" of London's layout drives structural brain changes. URL: https://www.ncbi.nlm.nih.gov/pmc/articles/PMC3268356/

28. Dresler M et al. (2017) Mnemonic training reshapes brain networks to support superior memory. URL: https://www.cell.com/neuron/fulltext/S0896-6273(17)30087-9?_returnURL=https%3A

%2F%2Flinkinghub.elsevier.com%2Fretrieve%2Fpii%2FS0896627317300879%3Fshowall%3Dtrue

29. Ackerman S. (1992) Discovering the Brain. URL: https://www.ncbi.nlm.nih.gov/books/NBK234146/

30. Kempermann G et al. (2015) Neurogenesis in the adult hippocampus. URL: https://cshperspectives.cshlp.org/content/7/9/a018812.full

31. Clive Wearing Wiki Page. URL: https://psychology.wikia.org/wiki/Clive_Wearing

32. Kim Peak Article. URL: https://www.wisconsinmedicalsociety.org/professional/savant-syndrome/profiles-and-videos/profiles/kim-peek-the-real-rain-man/

33. Coughlan S. (2015) Students 'cannot multi-task with mobiles and study'. URL: https://www.bbc.com/news/education-33047927

34. Brown AM & Kaminske AN. (2018) Five teaching and learning myths debunked: A guide for teachers. URL: https://www.taylorfrancis.com/books/9781315150239/chapters/10.4324/9781315150239-1

35. American Psychological Association (2006) Multitasking: switching costs. URL: https://www.apa.org/research/action/multitask

36. Weinschenk S (2012) The true cost of multi-tasking. URL: https://www.psychologytoday.com/us/blog/brain-wise/201209/the-true-cost-multi-tasking

37. Heng KWJ (2014) Teaching and evaluating multitasking ability in emergency medicine residents – what is the best practice? URL: https://www.ncbi.nlm.nih.gov/pmc/articles/PMC4306081/

38. Wallas, G. (1926). *The art of thought*. New York: Harcourt, Brace and Company.

39. Mental Chunking Wikipedia page. URL: https://en.wikipedia.org/wiki/Chunking_(psychology)

40. Memory Palace Blog Post. URL: https://medium.com/@freemededweb/memory-palaces-for-medical-students-7cafb4eae470

41. Zhang X & Bartol KM (2017) Linking empowering leadership and employee creativity: The influence of psychological empowerment, intrinsic motivation, and creative process engagement. URL: https://journals.aom.org/doi/abs/10.5465/AMJ.2010.48037118

42. Etymology of Avocado. URL: https://www.etymonline.com/word/avocado

43. Abbasi K (2011) A riot of divergent thinking. URL: https://www.ncbi.nlm.nih.gov/pmc/articles/PMC3184540/

44. Chase & Greg Memory Palace Podcast Episode. URL: https://medicalmnemonist.podbean.com/e/bonus-visual-markers-and-memory-palaces-with-chase-dimarco-interviewed-by-greg-rodden-of-physiology-by-physeo/

45. Anthony Metivier website. URL: https://magneticmemorymethod.samcart.com/referral/FREE-Memory-Improvement-Kit-97/im9TcwhnTZAMHkVj

46. Ryan Orwig Podcast Episode. URL: https://medicalmnemonist.podbean.com/e/memory-palaces-spaced-repetition-and-yoda-from-ryan-orwig-of-statmed-learning/

47. Alex Mullen and Cathy Chen Podcast Episode. URL: https://medicalmnemonist.podbean.com/e/memory-palaces-basics-w-mullen-memory-%e2%80%99s-alex-mullen-cathy-chen/

48. Staph aureus Wikipedia page. URL: https://en.wikipedia.org/wiki/Staphylococcus_aureus

49. Picmonic. URL: https://www.picmonic.com/my-picmonics

50. American Psychological Association (2009) The science of creativity. URL: https://www.apa.org/gradpsych/2009/01/creativity

51. Art of Memory, Dominic System. URL: https://artofmemory.com/wiki/Dominic_System

52. Art of Memory, Person-Action-Object (PAO) System. URL: https://artofmemory.com/wiki/Person-Action-Object_(PAO)_System

53. Witthoft N & Winawer J. (2013) Learning, memory, and synesthesia. URL: https://www.ncbi.nlm.nih.gov/pubmed/23307940

54. Key to Study, Hyperlinking technique. URL: http://www.keytostudy.com/personal-hyperlinking-format/

55. Davies M. (2011) Concept mapping, mind mapping, and argument mapping: What are the differences and do they matter? URL: https://link.springer.com/article/10.1007%2Fs10734-010-9387-6

56. Farrand P et al. (2002) The efficacy of the mind map study technique. URL: https://onlinelibrary.wiley.com/doi/abs/10.1046/j.1365-2923.2002.01205.x

57. Santiago HC (2011) Visual mapping to enhance learning and critical thinking skills. URL: https://journal.opted.org/articles/Volume_36_Number_3_VisualMapping.pdf

58. D'Antoni A et al. (2010) Does the mind map learning strategy facilitate information retrieval and critical thinking in medical students? URL: https://www.ncbi.nlm.nih.gov/pmc/articles/PMC2949690/

PART 4: SELF-ASSESSMENT

"Confidence comes not from always being right,
but from not fearing to be wrong."
Peter T. McIntyre

Congratulations on making it this far! We have covered a LOT of material in this relatively brief summary of the psychology of learning, education theory, and study skills. Knowing this stuff in theory is great, but it's not enough. Nor is aimlessly experimenting. Harkening back to our discussion of PDSA (plan, do, study, act), it's best to plan your actions ahead of time and self-assess on a regular basis. This helps to point your efforts in the right direction and ensure that you keep moving there. In this final section of the book, we will focus on self-assessment with a special emphasis on **Journaling**. We have mentioned the value of journaling throughout this book, but we have not covered its best practices in detail. Below we provide many examples of how you can use journaling for self-improvement. Pick something that works for your situation and adapt where necessary.

Journaling for a Better Life and Mind

Although most of us have had teachers and mentors recommend journaling at some point, it seems to be a tough habit to get going. There's no one-size-fits-all approach to journaling. There are general personal journals for keeping tabs of your daily thoughts and habits. There are gratitude journals that work on emotional self-reflection and cognitive-behavioral change. There are also memory journals for your mnemonics. If you simply type in "journaling" to a search engine, you'll find a plethora of approaches.

Though journaling has been historically celebrated for its cognitive effects, there are relatively few proper studies that illustrate its benefits. Journaling has been associated with decreased stress and improved memory [1] and reductions in depression severity [2]. It tends to provide an outlet to release anxiety and track your mental health [3].

Most research has been done on "expressive" journaling, where you recount your activities and feelings throughout the day, but we will provide other examples that are geared towards students. Whatever approach you choose, make sure your journals are kept in a secure space so you can feel free to *fully* express yourself.

For your Section Pre-tests

You may have noticed the **Pre-tests** throughout this book. You can use these by taking a baseline score and then retaking the pre-test at a later date once you've made some changes. All the items in the pre-test are tasks or strategies that can prime you to approach your studies more intentionally.

Do the pre-test questions help to identify your weak spots? How can you improve upon these weak spots? Do you use some of the suggested techniques and not others? Why? Keeping a journal for these pre-tests could be an easy way to begin regular self-assessment.

For your SMART Goals

When you set any significant goal, you should get into the habit of writing it down for later reference. So, you might as well record your goals in your journal! Ensure the goal is Specific, Measurable, Attainable, Relevant, and Time-bound. Having your goals recorded in this manner will give you an objective standard to live up to.

You can make an evolving list of short-term and long-term goals. Big goals could be updated on an annual basis, while smaller goals could be updated monthly or weekly. You could also photocopy these goals and place them on your wall (or equivalent) as a daily reminder.

For Habits

A habit tracker is a very simple type of journal that looks like a miniature calendar. Draw a small box that represents each day in the month. You won't write inside these boxes, so they can be very small. In a heading above the collection of boxes, write down the habit you wish to implement (or eliminate). Each day you meet your goal, mark its box with an X. It's that simple! You can easily keep a habit tracker for each new change you wish to make.

On days that you fail to meet your goal, take a moment to reflect on what stood in your way. Is there any way you could make changes to your environment that would facilitate or automate the habit? For example, if you have a bad Starbucks habit that's costing you too much money, you could take an alternate route to work/school to break the cycle of craving-stimulus-reward.

Note from Greg: Starbucks habit... guilty as charged.

For Work-Life Balance & Health Promotion

By using a journal to record your baseline mindset, physical activity, diet, sleep, and spiritual practice, you can quickly identify areas of strength vs. weakness. You may notice patterns in the data that can be acted upon to reinforce the good parts and eliminate the bad. Remaining oblivious about your own psychology is a sure-fire way to limit future growth.

Consider using the Experience Sampling Method to determine how you're feeling at any given point in the day. As we mentioned earlier in the book, the ESM is a validated tool that can help you to stop and take notice of your thoughts and feelings throughout the day [4]. You may notice particular pain points that can be eliminated or minimized where possible. Entire businesses are built around these kinds of insights where a keen observer identifies a pain point, comes up with a marketable solution, and charges for access to their services. Convenient access to ESM tools can be found on phone apps like PsyMate [5], which was developed by Maastricht University. Or if you'd like an analog version, see the Appendix.

For Happiness and Gratitude

There are many blogs written about how to create a Gratitude Journal. The American Psychological Association has a simple template, which we link to in the references [6]. It prompts users to spend about 15 minutes reflecting and expressing themselves to promote wellbeing.

UC Berkeley's Greater Good Science Center also has a few tips [7]. For example, an easy way to get started is to simply write down three things you are grateful for each day into your journal. If that doesn't appeal to you, consider using the Daily Mood Log developed by Dr. David Burns (a famous psychiatrist in the cognitive behavioral therapy movement) [8]. His log encourages users to identify their negative thoughts, then prompts you to identify any Cognitive Distortion that may have produced the negative thought. Becoming aware of the negativity - and its cause - makes it easier to recognize and avoid future negativity [9].

Whether you do this for your own happiness or for the sake of your future patients, it will be beneficial to try out a few of these exercises. Being *personally* familiar with them may be the best way for you to gauge whether your patient will respond.

For Study Sessions and Testing

Where should you focus your efforts? What are your weak points? We have covered numerous ways to answer these questions. In your journal, you should keep a record of your weak points and identify how you will remedy them. You could also keep track of your progress when trying out new tactics for your studies and exams, such as the MedEdge Method. To better prioritize your time, consider using our calculation from Part 2 that uses weighted averages to figure out where you can expect to gain the most points for your efforts. To supplement this, you could use the Covey Matrix or the Activity Based Costing chart from Part 1. Set aside a time each week to reassess and adjust your priorities. All of these activities can be done in a journal!

For Speed Reading

If you have decided to try out Speed Reading, write down your initial word-per-minute rate and monitor your speed over time. Alternatively, you could use something like the Habit Tracker app. How often will you do a training session and for how long? What is your comprehension rate after doubling your speed? Does the SQ3R method improve your comprehension? If not, does it depend on the type of material you are speed reading? All of these are important questions to consider. You can find a brief description of speed-reading journals at KeyToStudy.com [10].

For Visual Markers and Memory Palaces

In an interview, Dr. Anthony Metivier pointed out that a memory training journal ought to be structured in whatever way works best for you [11]. You can record lists of potential memory palaces, draw out diagrams of the palaces, record your Visual Dictionary for your visual markers, create your own Peg System or PAO System, or use it in any other way your creative juices see fit. Alternatively, you could draw out your memory palaces and mnemonics next to your class notes.

Remember that your sketches don't need to be works of art; they are meant to be a quick reference to fight the Forgetting Curve. A simple stick-man drawing may be sufficient to reignite the elaborate, dynamic visual mnemonic in your *mind's eye*!

For Diet

For those interested in personalized nutrition or weight loss, you could try keeping a food diary. While these are powerful tools, they can be time-consuming when done by hand. There are many apps available that make it easy to keep track of your food intake, like MyFitnessPal by Under Armour or MyPlate by Livestrong.

If you're testing out a new diet, consider monitoring how you feel after a week or two. But try to keep your observations objective. For example, record the amount of weight loss and the frequency of dyspepsia, constipation, diarrhea, heartburn, etc. Subjective measures of wellbeing, like your "mental clarity" or "energy levels," won't be of much help when you're scrutinizing the data.

Final Thoughts on Journaling

Now we have covered several methods for journaling, and the benefits that you may witness by making it a habit. All of these will have both short- and long-term utility. An interesting exercise would be to look back at some of your old journals from medical school when you become an attending physician, just to take a step back into your old self.

If you're looking for templates or other examples to get started, the Appendix contains useful resources. You could also try searching online for examples that more closely suit your needs. All of our updated templates and links can be found at FreeMedEd.org/MedStudent.

Concrete Examples to Guide Your Practice

Making Flashcards

Don't let anyone tell you medicine isn't about memorization. It is! Though conceptual knowledge is the ultimate endgame, this is not possible until certain terms, associations, and facts have been memorized. Using flashcards with spaced-repetition is a time-honored means to memorize information. However you decide to attack this, here are a few examples to guide your content creation.

When planning to create new study materials, it is important to know what resources are available to you. For example, Anki has pre-made flashcard decks that have been vetted by a huge number of medical students. These "community decks" are a great place to get ideas, but should not be exclusively relied upon. You should **consider making your own materials** that will help you to fill the gaps in your particular weak spots.

If you have access to recorded lectures or third-party educational videos, screenshotting important slides (and then inserting the image onto a digital flashcard) is an easy way to make high yield study materials. Online images, flow charts, tables, etc. also provide useful shortcuts for your flashcard answers. For hardcopy flashcards, you can simply write down the important points or print out the images.

On the front of the card, prompt yourself with **both open- and closed-ended questions**. This will require you to think critically and to know specific answers. For example, if you screenshot an image of the abdominal vasculature, you can make several related questions for the image. You could ask an open-ended question, like "Name each major artery/vein in the abdomen and what organ(s) they go to." Then, you could use the same flashcard to ask a closed-ended question, like "What arteries will a red blood cell travel through to get from the left ventricle to the spleen?" While it is much faster to do this with digital screenshots, you could also make these kinds of flashcards by hand (if you desire).

A few pearls about specific subjects: in pharmacology, you want to know about the drug's mechanism of action, *major* side-effects (i.e., Black Box warnings), and contraindications. In pathology, you want to know about the key pathophysiologic mechanisms of disease and any histopathologic buzzwords (which help you easily link the findings to the disease). Board examiners tend to avoid actually *using* these buzzwords in the vignette, so make sure you can convert a buzzword into more technical language.

For example, when you get a smear from a patient who has bacterial vaginosis, you would expect to see *Clue Cells* (buzzword for BV), but the technical description on the boards would look something like, "vaginal epithelial cells with obscure borders that are heavily coated by microorganisms." You'll also want to know what a clue cell looks like under the microscope.

In biochemistry, you'll want to know about rate-limiting enzymes and common diseases related to enzyme defects, such as glucose-6-phosphate dehydrogenase deficiency (G6PD). And in microbiology, you'll want to know about the basic features of the microbe. For example, with Giardia you'll want to know that it's a microscopic parasite that's usually ingested from dirty water, causes foul-smelling diarrhea, and can be treated with metronidazole.

One of the most difficult things for students to do at first is to create open-ended flashcard questions. These take time to write and to answer, which can be frustrating. But it would be a mistake to abandon open-ended flashcards! Optimal retrieval practice requires you to store, organize, and recall the information at the drop of a hat without any visual stimulus to guide you. Making your cards open-ended may seem daunting at first, but the benefits of working your brain *just a little bit harder* will start to accumulate with practice. Even if it takes 5 minutes to recall an entire flashcard, you are developing strong neural connections for later use.

When using open-ended flashcards, take one last-minute look at all of the facts you hope to recite, then close your eyes and start naming them off. You may be surprised by how difficult it is to recall information you were just looking at a few seconds ago! (You can use this recitation strategy for almost anything, not just flashcards.) After listing off everything you can remember, open your eyes and review the answers. Take note of the information you did not recall. Be honest.

It's easy to put information into a flashcard, assume you will recognize it next time, and push off the process of genuine self-assessment. This is the classic setup for the Illusion of Competence. Unfortunately, the Forgetting Curve is too harsh to ignore, so you need to keep up your skills with spaced repetition (see next section for details).

The point of these exercises is **to reduce cognitive load** during the test (and on the wards). Having certain facts and associations memorized will reduce the amount of mental energy you need to use in the moment of the exam (or when caring for your patient). For example, if you have put in the time to memorize (and chunk) the presentations of nephritic vs. nephrotic syndrome, then it just becomes an automatic habit to see the underlying pattern of nephritic vs. nephrotic in the vignette. So, instead of trying to decipher disparate signs and symptoms like hematuria, hypertension, and oliguria, you can just *instinctively know* that the patient has nephritic syndrome, and move on. By reducing your cognitive load in this manner, you can move through the question more efficiently to come up with the correct answer.

This kind of instinctive knowledge will also be helpful on the wards, but be careful not to jump to conclusions. You should always be able to explain your clinical reasoning in a step-by-step manner. That being said, it's a pretty good feeling when you're able to quickly recall information as your attending starts to "pimp" the students.

Spaced Repetition Schedule

To our knowledge, there's no consensus on the *optimal* spaced repetition schedule. It probably depends on factors like the type/difficulty of the material, your previous experience, and your academic goals. But from our experience, the **11311 Rule** tends to work well. Full disclosure: we don't have research studies to support this rule; it's completely anecdotal.

We recommend that you plan to see your first repetition of the material within 1 hour, then again in 1 day, 3 days after that, then 1 week, and at least once more at 1 month. To give you a better sense of what this looks like, we've made a sample spaced repetition calendar that you can download for free at our book page, FreeMedEd.org/MedStudent.

Unfortunately, it's hard to create this kind of customized schedule with a program like Anki, but you can experiment with the software and come up with a workable solution. Be warned, even though 5 Anki cards per day may not seem like much, the numbers add up. For example, by week 6, even if you get 100% correct answers, you'll be prompted with 25-30 cards per day. And incorrect answers will require even more repetitions. This gets to be overwhelming. Just remember, quality is more important than quantity for overall comprehension.

When it comes to flashcards, higher quality usually means higher difficulty. If you are making more difficult flashcards, such as having to recite an entire pathway from memory, it can take a while to get through all of your cards for the day. Despite this burden, we advocate for more open-ended cards than closed-ended cards because this mental recollection exercise potently reinforces memory (see previous sections for further explanation). It helps if you don't view flashcards as a simple/quick review, instead you should view them as an active learning exercise.

Question Banks and Simulated Study Sessions

In this last segment, we wanted to cover two very common mistakes medical students make when planning out their board exam review: 1) start their Qbanks too late; and 2) focus their efforts solely on Qbanks. Both of these mistakes will be costly. Let's take a look at how to avoid them.

Avoiding all Qbank questions until late in the game is common. First-year students often think they do not know enough information yet to answer board-style questions. Even though you'll get a bunch of questions wrong due to knowledge deficits, the purpose of Qbanks is NOT to get all the answers correct. It is to learn! Hence, you should incorporate Qbanks early on in medical school.

Initially, you should aim to become familiar with the style of board questions and you should identify your knowledge gaps (based on the material you've seen thus far, not the totally unfamiliar stuff). You should also figure out how long it takes you to thoroughly review a question, which includes reading and digesting the explanation for ALL the answer choices. Don't skimp on this part because it is critical! Most third-party Qbanks do a great job of providing solely high-yield material and leaving out the fluff. All of it will enhance your scores and your performance as a student doctor.

Another issue to be aware of is the overutilization of board-style Qbanks later in your studies. For instance, some students do not access top Qbanks until well into their second year and assume this is the *only* resource they will need. There are a couple issues here. First, if you haven't done enough questions leading into your dedicated study period, it will take a lot of effort to adjust to learning from Qbanks. Second, in order to finish the Qbank, you'll have many more questions to complete per day. For these reasons, we recommend that you incorporate Qbanks into your studies within the first half of your first year.

All that being said, don't sacrifice performance in your medical school classes to study for the boards. **Your classes should be the top academic priority.** If you fail your classes, you won't even have the opportunity to *take* the board exams.

Next Steps

As recommendations and resources may change in the future, we would ask you stay updated by following us on social medial and signing up for our newsletter. Or you can bookmark our page at FreeMedEd.org/MedStudent.

If you would like to engage with other readers of this book, you can share your ideas or pose questions to the community via our Medical Mnemonist Mastermind Group on Facebook. If you're interested in our podcasts, try searching for some of these: InsideTheBoards, Medical Mnemonist, Step 2 Secrets Podcast, Med School Phys, and Physiology by Physeo.

If you are currently starting clinical rotations, or know friends that are, consider getting advice from clinical educators via the 1-Minute Preceptor Podcast, and by using the FindARotation app to locate and schedule your own rotations across the country. More information can be found at FindARotation.com.

In closing, we hope you have enjoyed this book. Too often, important insights from fields like psychology, business, and wellness are completely overlooked during our medical education. We hope that you gained a few insights that will help to improve your studies, exam performance, and wellbeing.

If you found this material helpful, please reach out and let us know. We appreciate all feedback and comments! If you think this material would be helpful for your friends, classmates, or school, we hope you will share it with them. Contact us regarding potential Institutional Discounts on all FreeMedEd materials. Also, if you would like to be kept apprised on our future products, please subscribe to our email list at FreeMedEd.org and follow us on social media. See links below.

https://www.facebook.com/freemeded

https://twitter.com/FreeMedEd

https://youtube.com/freemeded

https://www.instagram.com/freemeded/

https://www.pinterest.com/freemeded/

References - Part 4

References can also be found at https://freemeded.org/book-references/

1. Carpenter S (2001) A new reason for keeping a diary: Research offers intriguing evidence on why expressive writing boosts health. URL: https://www.apa.org/monitor/sep01/keepdiary.aspx
2. Krpan KM et al. (2013) An everyday activity as a treatment for depression: The benefits of expressive writing for people diagnosed with major depressive disorder. URL: https://www.ncbi.nlm.nih.gov/pmc/articles/PMC3759583/
3. Walker SE (2006) Journal writing as a teaching technique to promote reflection. URL: https://www.ncbi.nlm.nih.gov/pmc/articles/PMC1472640/
4. Experience Sampling Method Wikipedia page. URL: https://en.wikipedia.org/wiki/Experience_sampling_method
5. PsyMate App. URL: https://www.psymate.eu/
6. Reed S et al. Lesson Plan: Practicing gratitude via a gratitude journal. URL: https://www.apa.org/ed/precollege/topss/teaching-resources/practicing-gratitude-lesson
7. Greater Good Science Center website. URL: https://greatergood.berkeley.edu/video/item/three_research_backed_tips_for_a_grateful_workplace
8. Daily Mood Log. URL: https://static1.squarespace.com/static/576754ecebbd1a42a8a816de/t/5a58f6d4f9619ab0c35897bb/1515779796871/Dailymood.pdf
9. Grohol JM (Updated 2019) 15 common cognitive distortions. URL: https://psychcentral.com/lib/15-common-cognitive-distortions/
10. Key to Study website. URL: http://www.keytostudy.com/using-reading-diary/
11. Anthony Metivier Podcast Interview. URL: https://medicalmnemonist.podbean.com/e/guide-to-memory-palaces-with-the-magnetic-memory-method-anthony-metivier-part-2/

Appendix

Active vs. Passive Learning Behaviors

Cognitively passive learning behaviors	Cognitively active learning behaviors
I previewed the reading before class.	I asked myself: "How does it work?" and "Why does it work this way?"
I came to class.	I drew my own flowcharts or diagrams.
I read the assignment text.	I broke down complex processes step-by-step.
I reviewed by my class notes.	I wrote my own study questions.
I rewrote my notes.	I reorganized the class information.
I made index cards.	I compared and contrasted.
I highlighted the text.	I fit all the facts into a bigger picture.
I looked up information.	I tried to figure out the answer before looking it up.
I asked a classmate or tutor to explain the material to me.	I closed my notes and tested how much I remembered.
	I asked myself: "How are individual steps connected?" and "Why are they connected?"
	I drew and labeled diagrams from memory and figured out the missing piece.
	I asked myself: "How does this impact my life?" and "What does it tell me about my body?"

Six Item Gratitude Questionnaire (GQ-6)

The Gratitude Questionnaire-Six Item Form (GQ-6)	
Using the scale below as a guide, write a number beside each statement to indicate how much you agree with it.	
1 = **strongly disagree**	
2 = **disagree**	
3 = **slightly disagree**	
4 = **neutral**	
5 = **slightly agree**	
6 = **agree**	
7 = **strongly agree**	
Questions	**Score**
1. I have so much in life to be thankful for.	
2. If I have to list everything that I felt grateful for, it would be a very long list.	
3. When I look at the world, I don't see much to be grateful for.	
4. I am grateful to a wide variety of people.	
5. As I get older, I find myself more able to appreciate the people, events and situations that I have been part of my life history.	
6. Long amounts of time can go by before I feel grateful to something or someone.	
Scoring Instructions	
1. Add up your scores for items 1, 2, 4 and 5.	
2. Reverse your scores for items 3 and 6. That is, if you scored a "7", give yourself a "1" and if you scored a "6", give yourself a "2", etc.	
3. Add the reversed scores for items 3 and 6 to the total from step 1. This is your total GQ-6 score. This number should be between 6 and 42.	

This assessment is a part of the public domain from the University of Miami.

Study Group Member Assessment

QUALITY	NAME	NAME	NAME	NAME	NAME
Respect: How much do you appreciate their values?					
Enthusiasm: How much energy to they bring to the meeting?					
Security: How safe do you feel sharing your ideas and thoughts with them?					
Reciprocation: How much do you grow each other's skills and knowledge?					
TOTAL					

Source: *Collaborative Intelligence* by Dawna Markova and Angie McArthur

Exam Grid Paper

EXAM GRID SIMULATOR

Name: _____ Date: _____

You can find a full page download at FreeMedEd.org/medstudent. Consider printing this page out and then laminating it. You can then reuse it with dry-erase markers. **How could you use the exam grid paper on the test?**

- Use the grid paper as a mental "dumping ground" at the beginning of your exam. Unload any mnemonics, difficult topics, or math equations so you don't have to remember them later.
- Use it solely to perform calculations.
- Use it as a space to conduct parts of our Basic Exam Technique or Tie-breaker Technique (or to write out the steps of these procedures).
- If you are artistic, you may consider drawing graphic representations that you have prepared for the exam, or even

Visual Markers you created (see Part 3 for more details about this). The less you have to remember under stress, the better! Also, these sketches don't need to be works of art, so long as you know what they mean. You are the only person who will see them.

Expansive List of Board Question Interrogatives

Basic Science Lead-ins
- Which of the following is the most likely cause/mechanism of this effect?
- Which of the following is the most likely causal infectious agent?
- This patient most likely has a defect in which of the following?
- This patient most likely has a deficiency in which of the following enzymes?
- Which of the following cytokines is the most likely cause of this condition?
- Which of the following structures is at greatest risk for damage during this procedure?
- The most appropriate medication for this patient will have which of the following mechanisms of action?

Obtaining and Predicting History and Physical Examination
- Which of the following factors in the patient's history most increased her risk for developing this condition?
- Which of the following additional information regarding this patient's history is most appropriate to obtain at this time?
- Which of the following is the most appropriate focus of the physical examination at this time?

Selecting and Interpreting Diagnostic Studies
- Which of the following is the most appropriate diagnostic study to obtain at this time?
- Which of the following laboratory studies is most likely to confirm the diagnosis?
- Which of the following is the most likely explanation for these laboratory findings?
- Arterial blood gas analysis is most likely to show which of the following sets of findings?

Formulating the Diagnosis
- Which of the following is the most likely diagnosis?
- Which of the following is the most likely working diagnosis?

Determining Prognosis/Outcome
- Based on these findings, this patient is most likely to develop which of the following?
- Which of the following is the most likely complication of this patient's current condition?

Health Maintenance and Disease Prevention
- Which of the following immunizations should be administered at this time?
- Which of the following is the most appropriate screening test?
- Which of the following tests would have predicted these findings?
- Which of the following is the most appropriate intervention?
- For which of the following conditions is this patient at greatest risk?
- Which of the following is most likely to have prevented this condition?
- Which of the following is the most appropriate next step in management to prevent [morbidity/mortality/disability]?
- Which of the following should be recommended to prevent disability from this patient's injury/condition?
- Early treatment with which of the following is most likely to have prevented this patient's condition?
- Supplementation with which of the following is most likely to have prevented this patient's condition?

Pharmacotherapy/Clinical Interventions and Treatments
- Which of the following is the most appropriate initial or next step in patient care?
- Which of the following is the most effective management?
- Which of the following is the most appropriate pharmacotherapy?

- Which of the following is the first priority in caring for this patient?

Mechanisms of Disease

- Which of the following is the most likely explanation for these findings?
- Which of the following is the most likely location of this patient's lesion?
- Which of the following is the most likely pathogen?
- Which of the following findings is most likely to be increased/decreased?
- A biopsy specimen is most likely to show which of the following?

*A more complete list can be found in Appendix B of the NBME Gold Book.

Post-Exam Autopsy Table

Post Exam Autopsy, Date:_____ Topic:_____

Question#	Correct Answer	Error Made	Reason for Error	Plan for Improvement

and % of each Error Type_____   # and % of Tie-breakers correct_____

Error Recording Scheduler

Error Recording Scheduler							
	Monday	Tuesday	Wednesday	Thursday	Friday	Saturday	Sunday
Negligence Errors							
1A							
1B							
1C							
Test Procedure Errors							
2A							
2B							
2C							
Conceptual/Study Errors							
3A							
3B							

Experience Sampling Method

Question/Statement	Scale	Rate Your Current Experience
I feel cheerful	1=not at all … 7=very	/
I feel insecure	1=not at all … 7=very	/
I feel relaxed	1=not at all … 7=very	/
I feel annoyed	1=not at all … 7=very	/
I feel satisfied	1=not at all … 7=very	/
I feel lonely	1=not at all … 7=very	/
I feel anxious	1=not at all … 7=very	/
I feel down	1=not at all … 7=very	/
I feel guilty	1=not at all … 7=very	/
(optional additional personal question)	Ex: happy, relaxed, stressed, angry, ashamed, etc.	
What am I doing?	Select: work or study, household, resting, eating/drinking, leisure, other, nothing	
I would rather do something else	1=not at all … 7=very	/
Where am I?	Select: at home, at family or friend's place, at work or school, public place, transport, somewhere else	
Who am I with?	Select: partner, family resident, family non-resident, friends, colleagues, acquaintances, strangers or others, nobody	
I am hungry.	1=not at all … 7=very	/
I am tired	1=not at all … 7=very	/
I am in pain	1=not at all … 7=very	/